"They Never Want to Tell You"

"They Never Want to Tell You"

Children Talk about Cancer

David J. Bearison

Harvard University Press
Cambridge, Massachusetts
London, England
1991

This book is printed on acid-free paper, and its binding
materials have been chosen for strength and durability.

Library of Congress Cataloging-in-Publication Data

Bearison, David J.
"They never want to tell you" : children talk about cancer /
David J. Bearison.
p. cm.
ISBN 0-674-88370-5
1. Tumors in children—Biography.
I. Title.
RC281.C4B43   1991
362.1'9892994'00922—dc20   90-49945
CIP
AC

Designed by Gwen Frankfeldt

In memory of my mother, Faye Soskin Bearison,
who, because of cancer, left me much too soon

Contents

*"The world breaks everyone and afterward
some are strong at the broken places."*

Ernest Hemingway

P*reface*

In her masterly essay *Illness as Metaphor,* Susan Sontag articulated the morbid obscenities that are culturally ascribed to cancer and the taboos constructed by our society to "protect" us from this disease. Like any cultural taboo, the notion of cancer (even the very word cancer) is to be avoided whenever possible except in metaphorical reference to the most heinous societal conditions. Yet every one of us will be profoundly affected in some way by cancer.

Growing up, we are socialized to implicitly abide by the insidious metaphors that are associated with cancer. However, when you listen to children who have cancer, you hear a different voice. The metaphors, clichés, and taboos have not been so firmly ensconced that the children hesitate to speak to us in a voice that exposes the culture of cancer and the conventionalized behavior and attitudes of those who function within that culture, as patients, cancer professionals, and families and friends. Listening to children talk about having cancer is a way of achieving Sontag's aim to strip cancer of its metaphors in search of a healthier way of being ill.

Initially, I intended a book that would help children who have cancer, but as I talked with more and more children, I began to appreciate that the issues they were advancing and how they were talking about them were not limited to children's concerns about having cancer. They are the concerns of anyone who has cancer, child or adult. The children were speaking in a voice that often was remarkably free of the social conventions, distortions, and defenses that adults use to hide similar questions and anxieties. By listening to children, we hear the voices of adults who have cancer speaking to us about issues that are not always as easy for them to articulate as they are for children.

Studies of child development historically have treated childhood as a period of profound developmental changes during which children acquire a variety of social and cognitive competencies on their way toward adulthood. From such a perspective, childhood is understood as a preparatory process in which adults have the responsibility to educate and socialize children. However, from another perspective, a perspective that is realized in the narratives of children who have cancer, childhood has its own values and competencies that are not less than the adults' but that are different. Thus, there can be times when adult ways of adjustment become inappropriate and when we can turn to children to find new ways of adjusting—ways that are more natural, maybe less "civilized," and not so cloaked in our collective and archaic fears, guilt, biases, and ignorance. Because of the rapidly changing climate regarding cancer and the search for new ways of coping with having cancer in our time and culture, it is necessary for us to listen to children speaking to us about their experiences and to learn and appropriate from them. Children speak to us in voices that are rich, compassionate, and honest. They are, therefore, our best narrators about the experience of having cancer. Thus, this book is not only about children who have cancer, it is about cancer as a human experience in its most profound sense.

My primary focus has been on the children's experiences because of my personal interest in child development and particular satisfaction in talking with children. But this book also focuses on the children's families and their treatment teams. From what the children say about their parents, siblings, and members of their treatment team, we can learn better ways for these individuals to talk with and listen to children—ways of talking and listening that will create a healthier and more comfortable climate for candid, sober, and enduring dialogues between children who have cancer and those that care for them.

What these children have to say about their experiences also is relevant to all children with severe chronic illnesses. Many of the continuing concerns of chronically ill children are reflected in what children have to say about having cancer, such as questioning why they are impaired when other children aren't; dealing with the reactions of their friends and families whose view of them as being different changes the ways in which children with cancer view themselves in relation to others; expressing their need for support from others while still maintaining their independence; adjusting to disruptions in the normal routines of growing up; and constantly struggling to understand their treatment and to find strength and meaning in their pain.

In 1981, when I first began to consider the special needs of children who have cancer, several studies had already confirmed that many of these children have serious adjustment problems during the two-to-three-year course of their treatment and often well beyond. However, the causes of their adjustment problems were not well understood. As a psychologist studying how children think, I was struck that there had been no studies of how these children thought about having cancer and how their thinking affected their adjustment reactions. Most of what was known about children's thoughts about illness was derived from studies of physically healthy children reflecting on hypothetical conditions of illness, instead of children for whom a life-threatening illness is a subjectively relevant, emotionally charged, immediately present, and prolonged experience to which they must continually adjust.

Children who have cancer are responding not only to the exigencies of treatment but also to their subjective understanding of their condition. How children are able to understand and make sense of their cancer experiences is a critical component in determining how they emotionally cope with them. Therefore, studying children's adjustments to having cancer without studying how they understand the experience of having cancer seemed like putting the proverbial cart before the horse. Consequently, I began studying how children who have cancer systematically construct and organize their knowledge about their illness and its treatment.

To gather data, I sent a research assistant to pediatric oncology clinics to ask children to describe everything that happens to them when they come for treatment. The children's responses were recorded and transcribed on a computer, and every single event that they described was coded, numbered, and statistically analyzed—what investigators refer to as "number crunching." As we were number crunching our data, I realized that we were losing the rich quality of what the children had been telling us. I remember talking about this with a clinical colleague, who compared it to plucking off the leaves of an artichoke but throwing away the heart.

After preparing these data-based studies for publication, I was determined to go back and recover the "heart." These children had been telling us a lot more than what we had been asking them. They welcomed the opportunity to talk about their experiences, and it seemed to be a way for them to give meaning to and make sense of their condition. Consequently, I undertook a clinical and ethnographic study of children's experiences of having cancer, as opposed to the previous data-based, number-crunching kind of study. This time, instead of sending a research assistant to the field to collect data, I personally met with the children and listened to them tell me what it was like to have cancer. Their stories, in their voices, are the focus of this book.

While preparing this book, I came to appreciate, as never before, my good fortune to be a member of a community of scholars at a university that promotes the freedom to explore new areas of inquiry in innovative ways. I am most grateful to my colleagues and students in the doctoral program in developmental psychology at the Graduate Center of the City University of New York, who graciously tolerated my spending so much time in different hospitals meeting with children and who acknowledged that there are other scientific methods in psychology besides experimental, data-based studies. Lauren Feinsot and Lea Kessler Shaw transcribed verbatim the audio transcripts and consistently remained true to the children's voices. The Rockefeller Foundation and Roberto and Geanna Celli provided me with an ideal setting and all the comforts of the Villa Serbelloni on Lake Como, Italy, in order to write.

There are several people to whom I am particularly grateful. They are Amia Lieblich of the Hebrew University of Jerusalem, who inspired me through her own books and through our friendship to go forward with what was for me a new form of inquiry; Irving Sigel, an extraordinary mentor and insightful founding editor of the *Journal of Applied Developmental Psychology*, who guided my previous publications in pediatric psychology; and Linda Granowetter, a dedicated pediatric oncologist, a special friend, and guide, who helped me to understand the children and their families from her exceptional perspective of care and professional expertise.

The physicians, nurses, psychologists, social workers, and

administrators at the pediatric oncology centers welcomed me without any reservations. They appreciated and supported the purpose of my project; they shared with me their knowledge and concern for the children; they allowed me to participate in their work and at times willingly worked around me; they helped me when I was feeling overwhelmed by it all; and they were my role models. In order to preserve the anonymity of the children, I regret that I can't mention these individuals and their institutional affiliations by name, but my sincere appreciation goes out to each individual among them.

My deepest gratitude goes to all of the children with whom I met and who welcomed me into their lives; who saw in me the opportunity to talk to others; who gave so willingly and openly; who showed such concern for and trust in what I was doing; and who wanted to be a part of my book. Some of them died, and I grieve and mourn their passing; others made remarkable progress and completed their treatment, and I share their sense of accomplishment and joy. I will never forget any of them. They taught me so much and made me a better therapist and a more caring person. Although I cannot mention them by name, I am sure they will recognize their stories in this book, and they will understand my gratitude.

D.J.B.
Villa Serbelloni
Lago di Como

Introduction

Talking with children

who have cancer

In the past twenty years, more effective kinds of chemotherapy, radiation, and surgery have produced remarkable
improvements in the course of cancer for most children. However, as prognoses for childhood cancer continue to improve
and survival times lengthen, the uncertainties associated with
having cancer are growing because surviving cancer in individual cases remains unpredictable. Adding to these uncertainties are undetermined and delayed toxic effects of increasingly complex treatment protocols. It is these uncertainties
with their life-threatening implications that constitute the psychological impact of having cancer. How children understand
and emotionally cope with such uncertainties during the prolonged course of their illness and well beyond is becoming
an important issue for those who treat and care for these
children.

Twenty years ago when the prognosis of childhood cancer
was dismal, how children adjusted to having cancer was not
an issue. The aim then was to make children as comfortable as
possible and to prepare their families for the process of griev-
ing. A common way of comforting children was to withhold
from them the diagnosis of cancer and the frightening knowledge of what such a diagnosis would entail. To do otherwise,
was considered cruel—a repudiation of any hope for recov-

ery, no matter how improbable. Only in recent years and only in certain cultures, including our own, has this practice begun to be displaced in pediatric oncology by the ethic of full disclosure between physician and patient.[1] However, this ethic is not easily defined.

Those who would argue that children always should be told the *truth* about having cancer must recognize that the truth is susceptible to many interpretations. How children understand what they are told about having cancer, how they ought to be told about it, and how it affects them at different phases of treatment and survivorship are critical questions that require careful and systematic examination.

Accepting the initial diagnosis of their child's cancer usually is the most difficult adjustment for parents.[2] They want to know what the probability is for their child's survival, as though knowing this will somehow help them gain some relief from their disbelief and shock. Consequently, this is what parents most often ask and expect from the physician upon learning that their child has cancer. Conveying the diagnosis to parents is also difficult for physicians, and, like parents, many of them resort to probabilities as a way of assuming a greater, yet false, sense of certainty in approaching the incredible uncertainties associated with having cancer.[3]

However, probabilities have very little meaning in individual cases; they are intended to denote group effects in experimental contexts. Any probability in an individual case is contingent upon a series of temporal and biological variables that have to be qualified by the rather absurd clause, "All other things being equal . . . " Of course, for any individual, all other things are never equal. During the protracted course of an individual child's illness, such probabilities may need to be revised. Relapses will lead to variations in treatment protocols which, in turn, will affect the child's biological reactions; the result will be a confusing series of mediated contingencies and uncertainties regarding ultimate progress.

Such kinds of truths, I would argue, are not helpful to children. They are not what children want to know about having cancer, and they generally will not help children to cope with having cancer. Thus, in place of probability statements, we need to consider how to inform children and their parents about having cancer and receiving prolonged treatment.

A prescription for informing children

Soon after learning about the implications of their child's diagnosis of cancer, parents must consider when and how to inform their child and if they want to be the ones to do so. The interim between when the parents find out about the diagnosis and when they feel ready to discuss it with their child is an unduly stressful time; the child's fears become exacerbated by carefully reading subtle cues and coming to understand that something is seriously wrong, no matter how well parents think that they can conceal this from their child. One little boy told me that he knew something was seriously wrong with him when, on the way home from the physician's office, his parents took him to a movie that he had been asking to see for weeks, then to his favorite restaurant, and then to buy him a special gift he had wanted. All the while his parents kept telling him how much they loved him and that nothing was wrong. His parents could not understand why their child showed no interest in the movie, had no appetite in the restaurant, and acted so blase about receiving a treasured gift. Later that evening, alone in his bed, the child was too frightened to fall asleep and too afraid to confront his parents. Parents' attempts to shield children from knowing the diagnostic implications of cancer do not alleviate their children's anxiety and fear. Instead, they escalate these emotions because children, even very young ones, simply are too good at reading between the lines. There probably is no greater anguish for children then to have no one with whom they can talk about their fear of being seriously ill because their parents are trying to protect them from the diagnosis of cancer. Sooner or later, these children inevitably will overhear hospital staff discussing their condition, and they also will find out about it from other children in the hospital. Not only will they become misinformed about their specific kind of cancer, but they will feel emotionally abandoned and will find it exceedingly difficult to trust those adults caring for them.

Because the treatment of cancer is complicated, uncertain, onerous, and protracted, children cannot be expected to tolerate it without understanding the nature of their illness and the need for their treatment. Children should be told about their diagnosis of cancer very soon after the parents' diagnostic conference with the physician. It is advisable that parents be with several members of the treatment team, particularly a pediatric oncologist, nurse, and child psychologist or pediatric social worker, when first informing children about the diagnosis and what their treatment will be like. In this way, questions that children have that might not have been anticipated by the parents or that might be too intimidating for them can be answered by members of the treatment team. Also, having members of the treatment team together with the parents conveys an impression to children that they are all there together to care for them and that they all share common knowledge and concern about what it is like for them to find out about having cancer. This will make it easier for children to share other stressful events both with their parents and with the treatment team as they inevitably will arise during the arduous course of treatment.

Often, when parents inform their child by themselves, circumstances are established whereby the parents continue throughout treatment to discuss issues with a physician or nurse with stipulations that their child not be told about them, and the child, in turn, discusses the same issues with stipulations that the parents not be told. This establishes an insidious process of concealment and mutual pretense between parents and child in which each deceives the other, thinking that by so doing they are making it easier for the other to cope. They end up saying the same things, expressing the same emotions, but never to each other.

During the diagnostic session, the psychologist or pediatric social worker can assess the emotional climate between parents and their child, assess how well they understand what they are being told, and advocate for their spoken and unspoken needs by questioning the physician and nurse, exploring different treatment options, and posing different reactions to what's being discussed. They also can assess the appropriateness of the parents' and child's reactions to learning about the treatment of cancer, define for them a normal range of adjustment, and propose appropriate kinds of psychological interventions.

The word "cancer" should not be avoided when discussing the diagnosis with children. They should be told in an age-appropriate manner what cancer is, in general, and in regard to their particular diagnosis. Terms such as malignant tumor, Hodgkin disease, and leukemia should not be used to mask the diagnosis of cancer because children will discover in other ways that they have cancer. For example, one child told me how he looked up the words "malignant" and "tumor" in a dictionary to discover that he had a life-threatening condition called cancer.

After parents, their child, and the treatment team has had the opportunity to meet, the treatment team should leave the parents and child alone together so that they can comfort one another. After a while, the treatment team again should meet with the child but this time without the parents present. At this meeting, the child should be made to feel that the treatment team is primarily there for his or her welfare and comfort and that their first commitment will always be to the child. The treatment team should also make it clear that the child is not expected to remember everything and that he or she is expected to ask a lot of questions during the course of treatment. Asking questions and talking should be encouraged, with the explanation that they are essential aspects of treatment.

In a manner consistent with children's level of development and cultural background, they should be told that they are seriously ill; that they will have to spend a lot of time in the hospital; that things probably will get worse before getting better; that because of the effects of treatment, they will most likely lose their hair but that it will grow back; that they will be able to talk with other children in the hospital who have cancer; that the people in the hospital are experts in treating their condition and have treated other children with the same condition; that treatment might continue for several years and that, at times, it might be very painful; that it's not possible at this time to predict when it will be over because of the possibility of relapses; that there will be various times when they will be scared and frightened; and that it's important to always ask questions, even very difficult questions like, "Am I going to die?" Children also need to know what interruptions to expect in their daily routines, such as attending school, participating in athletic events, and socializing with friends.

Parents and children usually will not take in all the information they are being told. They will forget most of it soon after their initial meeting and will act confused or even ignorant. This is a natural symptom of their emotional shock. Feelings of anger, fear, defeat, despair, resignation, inadequacy, helplessness, isolation, and passivity also are characteristic of the initial shock of a cancer diagnosis. In a few weeks, these feelings will begin to dissipate but then they will return to varying degrees at different critical phases of treatment.

Children need to appreciate that being scared and frightened is to be expected and that the best way to handle it will be to talk with people whom they trust. In the eyes of many children, as reinforced by their parents, "good" patients are strong, stoic, and brave and, in the words of one child, they take it like "a trooper." Our culture conveys the idea that the "good" patients are cured and the "bad" ones are not, and being good means being strong in the fight against cancer and being strong means not being afraid. Many of our cultural myths and metaphors about cancer convey the erroneous impression that we are not only responsible for contracting the disease but that we have the responsibility for fighting it and, thereby, curing ourselves.[4]

Thus, it is not uncommon to see parents admonish their children for crying or for expressing rage and fear in front of their physicians and nurses (and often I have counseled such parents that their child has a right to cry, to be afraid, and to be angry and that they, as parents, should not deny their child opportunities to express these emotions). The belligerent or rebellious patients who remain in touch with their anger and frustrations will be easier to deal with emotionally and will be more amenable to (and will be more likely to receive in the hospital) appropriate psychological interventions than the patients who struggle to deny these feelings. Although the former type of patients challenge the resources of their treatment teams, I am less worried about them then the so-called "good" patients who hide their frustrations, anger, and fears.

Children's psychological adjustment

As more and more children survive cancer, there is growing evidence that the experience of having cancer, receiving pro-

longed and arduous treatments, and coping with the enduring uncertainties of surviving cancer has profound and lasting
effects on children's psychological adjustment.[5] Children who
have cancer have a higher incidence of emotional stress and
adjustment problems than children who have other kinds of
chronic but not life-threatening illnesses.[6] Furthermore, as the
duration of treatment increases for most chronically ill children, their levels of anxiety decrease, while the opposite
occurs for children with cancer.[7] In addition to the stresses of
having cancer, the stresses of long-term cancer survivorship
also have been shown to be associated with significant psychological and social adjustment problems.[8]

What children know about their condition, their need for
treatment, and its painful consequences has been shown to
significantly affect how they adjust to having cancer. Children
who are told about having cancer early in their treatment are
better able to cope than children who indirectly learn about
their cancer later.[9] However, regardless of what, how, and
when they are told, children who have cancer, even very
young ones, are able to gather enough incidental cues from
parents, peers, siblings, and medical staff to realize that their
condition is serious enough to be life-threatening. Children
who have cancer actively struggle to organize and make
sense of their experiences. Often, they display a seemingly
precocious discernment of the medical procedures, the
biomedical implications of sequentially more toxic forms of
chemotherapy, and the prognostic consequences of relapses
following progressively briefer periods of remission.

Although there is an impressive array of experimental data
and psychological theories regarding normal childhood development, very little is currently known about what constitutes
a "normal" or adequate range of adjustment reactions among
children to stress and trauma.[10] This is a formidable problem
in understanding children's reactions to cancer. Although

children with cancer confront a frightening array of emotionally and biomedically stressful events, normal developmental processes are unfolding in spite of their illness. Thus, children's adjustments to having cancer unfold within the dimensions of normal development as well as within the atypical course of development occasioned by cancer. Basic developmental processes occur in synchrony with the stresses of having cancer. Children with cancer, not unlike healthy children, have needs for achievement, affection, and peer relationships. Opportunities for them to gratify these fundamental developmental needs will facilitate their adjustment to having cancer as they struggle to achieve some sense of normalcy in their lives.[11]

Creating a climate for talking

What issues should be considered when trying to establish and maintain a candid yet supportive dialogue with a child who has cancer? First, we need to discern when to talk with a child and when not to. It is a mistake to think that through our love and concern for a child who has cancer we can assume his or her burden and suffering. Although every child affected by cancer belongs to a family that shares their child's anguish, every child ultimately is alone in his or her struggle with cancer. While we can explore ways of helping children in that struggle, we cannot deny them the struggle nor the integrity of confronting it in their own way, no matter how young they are. Therefore, we need to learn how to recognize the signs and respect the limits and distance a child places between self and others at different times and to varying extent without imposing our own limits and distance on the child. This is not easy and, often it can be very painful to do so. While we may want to fuse ourselves with a child, we have to learn when to stand apart and give the child his or her own space to cope.

Also, we need to recognize our own fears about confronting the issues of cancer and how we unwittingly convey these fears to children. It is not the children who are unable to tolerate hearing about the painful consequences of having cancer but the parents and physicians who often cannot tolerate telling the children the consequences. Children's reluctance to talk about their condition reflects the anxiety and tension that they perceive in others more than their own anxiety. Children who have cancer become masters at perceiving what others are reluctant to talk with them about. When these children decline to talk about their condition in the presense of adults, it does not reflect their lack of concern or their innocence but their sense that adults are unable to talk candidly about it.[12]

During the course of their treatment, children come to understand how their parents and staff members expect them to behave and what they want to hear from them. In order to maintain their presumed impression of what it means to be a "good" patient and a "good" son or daughter, children often establish an elaborate set of behaviors that they unwittingly follow in order to maintain a mutual pretense with others that their condition is not so serious as to be life-threatening and that their complete recovery is imminent.[13] This kind of mutual pretense and conspiracy of silence between adults and children is not limited to having cancer. It often is enacted around other kinds of childhood traumas, including the death of a parent or a sibling, parental divorce, and child abuse.

If and when children's concerns about their treatment and prognoses become forbidden topics of discussion with adults, they become unremitting topics of discussion with other children who have cancer. By carefully and systematically reading subtle cues around them and by sharing information with other children who have cancer, children inevitably will find ways to learn about their illness when such knowledge is not openly accessible to them. Consequently, there is no valid reason to believe, as we did in the fifties and sixties, that we can possibly "protect" children from unnecessary anguish by not openly discussing with them the sober consequences of having cancer.

The need for supportive care

The increasing specialization of medical practice has created unique and essential roles for psychologists and pediatric social workers in the treatment of children who have cancer. The stereotype of a benevolent physician who takes care of everyone, listens to everyone's problems, and administers as much sympathy as medication seems lost, if it ever really existed. Today, physicians are perceived as medical experts who rely on a vast array of drugs, diagnostic procedures, and technologies to make their treatment decisions. The depersonalizing of medicine and the perception of the physician as a kind of "medical engineer" are not consistent with a view of the physician as someone who is there to help patients talk about their feelings and cope with the stresses of serious illness.[14] Many patients feel that talking about such things with a physician, particularly a specialist like a pediatric oncologist, interferes with the physician's work and, consequently, might jeopardize the quality of care they receive. Thus, many people feel that they have to enact the role of the "good" patient for the physician by not expressing emotions, by hiding their anxiety and distress, and by not questioning treatment procedures.

Many pediatric oncologists cringe at the thought of being perceived this way by their patients because they appreciate the risks and uncertainties associated with treating cancer and the emotional impact it has on children. They want to administer to the full range of their patients' needs, both emotional and biological. However, I do not think this is possible. I first realized this when I asked pediatric oncologists what they tell their patients about treatment procedures. All of them told me that they never perform a procedure on a child without first explaining what they are going to do. However, when I asked them what they said when a child questioned why they were going to perform a particular procedure, the physicians told me that children hardly ever questioned their procedures. After observing several of them perform procedures, I discovered that the way they spoke to children, although very benevolent, conveyed the message that the physicians were not there to discuss medical practice with their patients and that, understandably, it was not a matter for the children to negotiate whether or how a procedure was to be performed. Also, because many procedures, such as a spinal tap, are very painful, it is exceedingly difficult for children, particularly very young ones to reconcile the benevolence of a physician with the pain that he or she is inflicting upon them. These are all legitimate reasons, behaviorally and culturally conditioned, for children to feel threatened and intimidated by pediatric oncologists. Therefore, pediatric oncologists, while sensitive and responsive to the emotional needs of their patients, must also recognize the function of less threatening members of their treatment teams.

Psychologists and pediatric social workers are perceived by the children within the institutional context of the hospital as individuals who, despite their close comradery with physicians and nurses, do not participate in the practice of medicine and do not make what the children sometimes perceive to be life-or-death decisions about them. They are the "talk" and "play" doctors who, by talking and playing with children, help them deal with their feelings. This professional role is implicitly recognized by the children in their active struggle to make sense of their condition and to learn how to emotionally adjust to it.

I see this attitude among children with whom I meet for weekly psychotherapy sessions. When, for example, I see four- or five-year-olds in play therapy, I am always somewhat baffled by their benign willingness to put up with the disruption of their normal routines to make the trip to my office for fifty minutes to play with what to them must seem like an old man who often acts more like a foolish child. I play with them but only on a certain day, and I am always insistent that it can be only for a very limited amount of time. Outside of these limits, I never see them or talk to them; it is not a natural kind of relationship. And yet these children, who continually question me about a thousand things in their lives, never question me about who I am and what they are doing here with me. They don't because they come to appreciate, in ways they could never verbally articulate, that through their play with this person they are getting help in resolving their problems— problems that are too complex and emotionally painful for them to resolve on their own. In the same way that young children come to appreciate the value of play therapy, older children and adolescents come to appreciate talk therapy.

With more encouraging prognoses associated with childhood cancers and the uncertainties in individual treatments, it has become increasingly important for children to have psychologists and pediatric social workers on their treatment teams with whom they can talk and play. It is testimony to the remarkable medical progress we have achieved in treating childhood cancers that we are now able to turn our attention to ways of assisting children to cope emotionally with having and surviving cancer.

Telling their story

The purpose of this book is to illustrate the variety of ways in which children who have cancer feel comfortable talking about their experiences. The illustrations are in the form of narratives using the children's own words and dialects so that the reader will be able to hear how the children speak and what issues they choose to speak about. A narrative is a story consisting of a series of characters, settings, and events that are structured according to the perspective of a particular storyteller. In the present context, each child with whom I met was a different narrator, and the narratives were about what it is like to have cancer.

I met with more than 75 children at several pediatric oncology centers. These meetings could only have occurred in centers that discuss the diagnosis of cancer with children, a practice that is the norm in this country but not in many other countries. In general, I think I had access to children who were more open and comfortable talking about their cancer experiences than most children. In only two cases was I asked not to use the word "cancer" during my meetings with children because it had never been used by their parents or staff in front of them, at their parents' request. However, in both cases the children spontaneously used this word with me when describing their condition.

In considering how many children to see and how long to keep seeing them, I was guided by how well their narratives captured the phenomenological experiences of all children who have cancer. Accordingly, I continued meeting with children until I sensed that I had heard it all and felt it all and that listening to another child would not have added anything to what had already been expressed by the other children, although each child had a unique way of expressing his or her experiences.

To get the children's permission to talk with them and record what they were saying, I simply told them that I wanted to write a book about how children talk about their experience of having cancer so that others would better understand what it was like for them. Many children told me they wished that there was such a book they could have read when they found out they had cancer, or that they could have given to their family and friends to read. Also, many children said that they wanted members of their treatment team to read such a book about their experiences. All of them felt that talking with me would be a way of helping other children who have cancer, and this sense of caring and helping other children was very important to them.

The children ranged in age from three to nineteen years and represented a full compliment of economic classes and a variety of ethnic backgrounds—Afro-Americans, Caucasians, Hasidics, Hispanics, and Asian-Americans. They had all of the common forms of childhood cancers (with the exception of cancers of the central and sympathetic nervous systems), including leukemias, Hodgkin disease and other lymphomas, and solid tumors such as osteogenic sarcoma, Ewing sarcoma, rhabdomyosarcoma, and Wilms tumors.

Different children were seen at different phases of treatment, from the initial diagnosis to the conclusion of treatment and periodic monitoring of progress off treatment. Some children were seen only once, while others were seen several times, typically at critical times in their illness, such as a relapse, surgery to remove a tumor or limb, or when approaching death. All of the children were seen alone when I was recording what they were saying to me. Parents and staff were never present. In a few cases I met with two children talking to each other about their experiences.

I explained to the children that what they said to me would be confidential in the sense that it would not be repeated to their parents or other children. However, I also explained that there might be times when, unless they explicitly requested otherwise, I would share certain things that they said with the pediatric oncology staff. This occurred when I heard things that led me to think that a child had seriously misunderstood a medical procedure, had a legitimate grievance with a member of their treatment team but was reluctant to talk directly with him or her about it, was in emotional distress or feeling suicidal, was seriously violating medical compliance, or was generally acting self-destructively outside the hospital setting. Such pernicious behaviors included drug and alcohol abuse, unprotected sexual activities, reckless athletic activities, and failure to self-administer medications. I also would have shared information with the staff if I had reason to believe that any child was receiving other than appropriate care from any member of any treatment team. However, I never found this to be the case. On the contrary, I was continually impressed by the quality of care that all of the children received.

The children were told that they could request that I turn off the audio recorder or terminate our meeting at any time (although no child ever did). They also were told that their names would not be revealed in any publications and that all reasonable precautions would be taken to preserve their anonymity. For many of the children, this was a great disappointment. They wanted to be identified and be known. They had a strong sense of pride about themselves and the contributions they could make in helping others.

The children were seen when they were either hospitalized or visiting an out-patient pediatric oncology clinic. I felt that it was important to establish a role for myself as part of the treatment teams of attending physicians, research fellows, clinical fellows, nurses, social workers, and administrative assistants by being a participant observer. Thus, I sometimes attended case conferences, accompanied physicians on patient rounds, met individually with some of the members of the treatment teams, and sometimes was present when parents and their children first learned about the diagnosis of cancer. Also, I hung around in the out-patient clinics and hospital wards. In the clinics, my station was usually in the physicians' consultation room and in the patients' play/waiting room, where I sat at the tables with the children in order to participate in their play and listen to them talking among themselves. In the hospital wards, I hung around the nursing station where many of the children gathered and visited them (with their permission) in their rooms.

Sometimes I watched television with them, played board games with them, and talked to them about sports, school, and things they did with their friends and siblings. Sometimes we gossiped about other children and about some of the staff. During these informal meetings our conversations were not recorded. In these ways, I became a familiar fixture to the children—someone with whom they could easily talk, someone who was writing a book about them, and someone who, like the members of their treatment team, genuinely cared about them and wanted to help them.

The clinical method

The general approach I used to elicit narratives from the children about having cancer is known as the clinical method. My particular approach also had certain affinities with two other research methods in the social sciences, ethnography and phenomenology. In ethnography, the investigator, usually an anthropologist, enters a foreign culture as a participant-observer for the purpose of systematically describing the social environment from the native's point of view. In phenomenology, the investigator tries to capture a holistic construction of some behavioral phenomenon by capturing individual accounts in order to arrive at a common, universal account with as few presuppositions, biases, and prejudices as possible.

The hallmark of the clinical method is the way the investigator interacts with participants in order to maintain and follow their own lines of reasoning about their experiences. It is very different than conducting an interview using questions to elicit answers about predetermined issues that interest the investigator. Instead, questions and comments are used as a means of encouraging participants to elaborate on issues and events they deem relevant. Because questions and comments have not been prepared in advance and standardized, the investigator must continually remain within the psychological space of each participant in order to know when and how to probe further in a nondirective manner.

The investigator also must be aware of and monitor his or her own biases and prejudices about what he or she is hearing so as to hold them in suspension, as much as possible, from the interaction. The kinds of questions and probes used by the investigator are designed to acknowledge and give credence to each participant's idiosyncratic modes of verbal expression and discourse, rather than suggesting topics or providing interpretations. Thus, participants are encouraged to spontaneously raise issues that they feel are important to talk about, and to remain true to the variety of ways in which they feel comfortable talking about them.

A critical aspect of the clinical method is the assumption of unconditional positive regard—whatever a participant says is accepted without judgment. Positive regard is conveyed by maintaining eye contact, by showing acceptance through facial and body cues, and by generally indicating that you are with him or her and listening carefully. The expression of positive regard is effective only when the various channels of communicative responsiveness are synchronous with one another. For example, a child might express attitudes and opinions or describe behaviors of which I might personally disapprove. If I communicate acceptance at one level by eye contact and positive head nods while at another level I communicate disapproval by tightening my body posture and wincing at the corners of my mouth, the contradiction will be detected by the child, and accordingly the child will have more difficulty being candid with me. Because it is not possible to continually monitor every one of our communicative channels, unconditional positive regard is not so much a technique as an attitude. It derives from a commitment to accept children as they present themselves and not try to judge or change them—to learn from them instead of the other way around, which is the more typical arrangement in adult-child relations.

An attitude of unconditional positive regard is designed to give children complete freedom to talk about anything. However, it is not a natural attitude that parents would want to assume with their children, or physicians with their patients. Parents and physicians have certain responsibilities for the welfare of children in their care, and therefore they cannot unconditionally accept anything that children say or do. They have the responsibility to make judgments and distinguish inappropriate and self-destructive behaviors from appropriate and self-enhancing behaviors.

In my meetings with the children I could not assume a thoroughly dispassionate position, and there were times when I compromised the standards of the clinical method. For example, when I felt that children were needlessly blaming themselves for having cancer, I talked about how we do not really know the causes of cancer in children and that it could not possibly be from anything that they had said or done. When children's descriptions of a medical procedure or condition seemed grossly distorted, I discussed the procedure with them and suggested that they discuss it further with their physician or nurse. However, I also was sensitive about when to intrude on children's ways of perceiving a procedure or condition and when to accept them as part of a process of "healthy" denial. For example, the evening before surgery to remove a tumor, a child told me how the surgery was going to "cure" him by "removing the cancer from my body." This was not quite the case: if it had been, then why would he have to continue on a two-or-three-year regimen of chemotherapy? But this way of thinking about the surgery helped this child cope with his fears. He persuaded himself that, although the risk was great, the benefits were greater, and then it would all be over. After the surgery, the child would come to understand that it is not all over, and he might construct other kinds of denials to deal with future risks.

Children use different kinds of denials as defenses against their anxieties about having cancer. These unconsciously constructed denials help them defend against fears which, if left undefended, would be emotionally overwhelming. They are unconscious in the sense that the children do not think about different ways to defend themselves against fears about which they are consciously aware, and they are not aware of how they are distorting their perception of events in the service of denying them. When such denials become so great that children are unable to accept the vicissitudes of having cancer and consequently thwart their treatment by not complying with procedures, or when they become reluctant to admit to any fear or uncertainty about having cancer, their defenses are detrimental and need to be diminished. Some degree of fear and anguish must come to consciousness in order for children to recognize the seriousness of their condition so that they will recognize the need to comply with formidable treatment, abide the pain and toxic side effects, understand how others are responding to their condition, and accept their need to talk about it.

Another form of defensive denial is verbally stating the opposite and thereby negating the fear. This typically is expressed repetitively and somewhat out of the context of what else is being said. For example, one child kept repeating in different contexts and in different ways, "I know I'm not going to die," "Not that I feel that I'm going to die, but . . . ," "I'm really very, very, very sure that that's not going to happen." In this way this child was denying his fear of dying. As children become more comfortable talking about having cancer, many of their denials begin to dissipate, and they become better able to cope with acknowledged fears and uncertainties.

In a similar manner, I had to be sensitive to the children's use of ambiguous expressions, particularly in regard to issues that were emotionally threatening for them. All children, to varying extent, are egocentric in that they assume that because they know the referents to expressions they use, their listener does also. Thus, they are less likely than most adults to monitor their speech from the perspective of their listener in order to ensure that they are being properly understood. When in doubt about what a child meant, I would ask him or her to explain further. For example, a child told me, "I was really scared of *that*," and "I didn't want to think about *that*." In the context of what else she had been talking about, the word "that" could have referred to death and dying, and it might have been less anxiety provoking for her to refer to death and dying by using an ambiguous pronoun. But when I asked her what she meant by "that" she told me it had to do with going to a hospital. Now, one can imagine that children's expressions about fears of death and dying might have had greater dramatic impact for someone writing a book about having cancer than their fear of being hospitalized, but for me to have assumed that the child was speaking about death and dying without questioning its ambiguous expression would have been as egocentric for me as a listener as it had been for the child as speaker.

The ambiguity in children's speech, together with their reluctance to speak to us about experiences that they know make us uncomfortable, encourage adults to project on to children our own fears about cancer. We are reluctant to ask them to be more explicit, because we think that doing so will make it more painful for them, and also because it will be more painful for us to hear them talk about what we ourselves fear. Consequently, we allow and even encourage their ambiguities in order to maintain distance from them as a way of protecting ourselves. In parallel, our speech to children who have cancer can become filled with verbal ambiguities that hide our own fears. Children, recognizing our reluctance to talk explicitly with them about cancer, in turn augment their natural tendency for ambiguous speech in order to maintain a kind of mutual pretense with others in accordance with what they perceive others are emotionally able to hear.

Denial and the use of ambiguous expressions, as well as other kinds of defenses, occur reciprocally in the continuing interaction between children who have cancer and adults who talk with them about the experience. Often, both children and adults need help in overcoming their defenses, in order to establish and maintain a meaningful and honest dialogue.

About this book

The focus of this book is on the narratives of eight children who have cancer. These particular narratives were selected because they were some of the most expressive and revealing of the diversity of issues voiced by all of the children, but not necessarily because they were the most dramatic or heart-rending accounts. They encompass the full range of children's concerns. The narratives have been edited to delete my questions, probes, and comments and to organize the children's discourse in a nonrepetitive temporal sequence. This type of editing was minimal in that my questions, probes, and comments did not have the effect of eliciting topics, and for the most part the children spontaneously organized their thoughts in temporal sequence. This is a natural format for talking about one's experiences.

Every word in each narrative is the child's own, expressed in his or her own dialect. Each narrative is derived from a single child, that is, narratives from several children were not combined to form a composite narrative. The children's names have been changed and the names of attending staff, when mentioned, have been deleted and replaced by their professional titles. The diagnoses of the eight children have not been identified because what they have to say about having cancer is not particular to any specific kind of cancer. Also, the children are not identified by age or economic or cultural background for a similar reason, although this kind of information often is apparent in their narratives.

Following the narratives are eight themes that are common among almost all children who have cancer. These themes are illustrated with material from my meetings with children other than those eight whose narratives form the core of this book.

The primary purpose of the narratives and themes is to familiarize readers with the rich variety of ways in which children talk about having cancer, so that it will be easier for them to talk openly and honestly with children (as well as adults) about the experience of having cancer. For those who have cancer, reading these narratives will help them to better appreciate that they are not alone with their thoughts and feelings. I often sensed that the children with whom I met were talking more to others who have cancer (both children and adults, as well as to themselves) than to any other group of people and that, accordingly, I served simply as a conduit for their discourse.

While there might be a nagging temptation to interpret the children's narratives and to try to distinguish those that might reflect an adequate adjustment from those that do not, I advise against this. Instead, simply listen to the children speaking in their own voices about issues and events that are important to them. There is a great deal to be learned and appropriated from their narratives. They teach us the value of listening to children on their own terms without judging them so that their internal voices will become louder in our time.

*T*he narratives

You're still the same old Ant to us

Well, it started in September. I went that summer to Puerto Rico, and when I was there towards the end of my vacation my aunt noticed that I had like a lump on my back, so she called to New York and told my mother about it. At first it was like small, it was like a little mosquito bite so I let it slide, then after, she called again, and said it's bigger now, like the size of a lemon. By the next week, it got like a handful so my mother said, "Come back to New York 'cause I'm gonna have the doctor check you out." So then I went to this local hospital and then they told my mother that they were gonna send me to this hospital so they could run tests on me. So I came over here and they did tests, they did a biopsy and all that. Then they told my mother and they finally told me that I had cancer, and that I had to get an operation, and after the operation I would get radiation, and after that I would get chemotherapy for like a year.

The first time they told me I was like, "I got cancer, check that out." I was like shocked, and yet I wasn't angry or nothing. I was like, "We'll do whatever it is, I'm sure that it will be alright." So they did the operation and everything was a success and then they gave me chemotherapy and radiation. I was on it all this time, and then in the spring of this year, I was in remission, 'cause I was finished, all of spring, April 'til

June, when it started again and they told me that it came back again.

Then it hit me. The fact that my hair grew back and I was like crazy about getting it over with. I thought, "Damn, another year without hair and going through life." And it really got to me. I was like, "Oh no, my hair!" That was the thing that I was most scared about then. 'Cause in school, nobody really bothered me, but I felt it. Like in class everybody had to take their hat off, but I had permission to keep my hat on. All the guys used to look at me like why he could keep his hat on and all of this. A few of the guys that I was close to knew about it, but not in all my classes and I wasn't close to everybody.

It wasn't hard to tell them 'cause they asked me how come I was away for like six weeks. They was like, "What happened to you?" Since the teachers knew, they told the class. Then the guys like they said, "I heard that you had an operation" and all this, and so I told them. The teacher let us have one period like a little conference between me and my friends. She asked me like who I wanted to talk to, this was during the lunch period, so she took us to this little room and then told me to tell them. So, I told them, "Look guys, I'm not the same as I was before 'cause I got cancer now." They was shocked, they was like, "You got cancer! You, out of all people. Why it's you? You're a good guy." And I was like, "Well, you know, it's just some people get it, some don't." They felt bad for me, and I was like, "Yo, don't worry about it." And they asked me, "Is it real bad, are you gonna make it?" I told them, "Don't worry about it, I'm gonna make it. They gonna give me therapy, and give me radiation," and I talked about it.

This was before my hair fell out. I told them in a couple of months my hair's gonna fall out and I'm gonna go bald, then my friend Chris, I'll never forgot this, he say, "Yo, don't worry about it, you still the same old Ant to us." I felt real good when he said that, and he said, "I'm not gonna change. You're still gonna be my best friend." And he was like, "Don't worry. And if anybody makes fun of you, 'cause you lost your hair or something, you let me know, 'cause I'll talk to that person." He was real understanding, all the guys I told they felt bad. Nobody closed me out, and when we got angry, there were times that we would argue and I would think that maybe they would get mad at me and bring that up and start bothering me about it, but they never did, no matter what the reason why they got angry, so it was real good.

I have several friends that wanted to ask me about my sickness but they didn't know how to ask me because they was afraid to ask me because they didn't know how I would react. Like my neighbor, at first she didn't know how to come up to me. She wasn't sure if she should just ask me, "How do you feel about your sickness?" because she didn't know how I would react, and then one day, she spoke to a friend of mine that she knew was close to me, and she told him that she wanted to talk to me, so my friend told me, so I went to her house, and I brought it up, and that's when she told me that she didn't know how to say this to me, and the reason she didn't come out earlier was because she was afraid. Then I got close to her and we became the best of friends. I brought it up and I told her not to worry, that I wasn't afraid to talk about my sickness and then she asked me about it.

This one person asked me, um, "Can you catch it?" Like, "How did you catch it?" and this sort of stuff. And I said, well, I told the person, "Well, cancer you really can't catch it. But it's like, it's something that grows in your body over years, it develops." Like you really can't catch it, 'cause this person asked me, you know, "How did you catch it, could you have avoided catching it?" And I was like, well, no, you couldn't have, 'cause there was no way of knowing. And it's something that just grew over years. Some guys they would ask me, "Could I catch it from like," you know, like, they said, "like from drinking out of the same cup as you or something?" And I was like, "No you can't catch it."

When it relapsed, I felt bad, and I'm not ashamed to admit it, but I cried a little that night. I thought, "All over again, I gotta go through this." And then I figured, "Hey, I might as well keep fighting because it worked the first time, it will work the second time, and I'm gonna fight it, I'm not just gonna sit there and let it lick me." At times, when I get the chemo, I get sick, and you know, I feel bad because I already know, because I've been through it already, and just the fact of knowing that you gotta go through it all over again, all the being sick, throwing up, and everything about it, just made me feel real bad.

The doctor says that he's trying some new medicine that's a lot stronger. When he first started he said, "Don't worry about it," and I asked him, "Doctor, tell me straight out, I could take it, do I have a chance or what? Tell me the truth." And then he was frank with me. He told me that there was still a lot of medicines out, and they were going to try radiation, and as a last resort, he would do an operation. So he said, "Don't worry, you still got a chance." And he told my mother that. My mother told him, "Tell my son everything because he has the right to know," and a lot of times my mother didn't want to be the one to break the news to me because she felt bad that she had to say it, let alone live with it. So the doctor would tell me, and I take it like a trooper. I tell him, "Be straight up with me," and he tells me straight up. He said, "I can't promise you anything, but we'll see how the medicine works, and I'll give you tests and all that."

But with some people, not that they shouldn't be straight up, but with some people, it's like, they gotta tell it to them differently. Because if they come straight out, that person might not take, you know might not be as strong-minded and be able to take it, but I always told the doctor, "Be straight with me," and "I'm a strong person so you really won't, won't offend me." And I'd rather have it like that than, you know, find out another way. All my friends, as far as I know, they'd rather have the doctors come straight up and tell them what's going on. And in a way, I think it's good that the doctor should tell all his patients everything straight up, 'cause sooner or later the patients gonna find out another way and then, I think, it'd be worse.

Like you're not supposed to, according to the nurses, a patient's not supposed to go into his chart and look through it. Well, but there are some patients that once in a while, they get a little curious and want to know a little more than they already know. 'Cause sometimes there's nobody at the nurses' station and it's unattended and they may see their chart there, and you know they may want to look at it. 'Cause, of course, it has their name, so they could read it. There's nothing wrong with that. And you know, I figure that they'll find out something that they shouldn't find out just yet, and not the way that they read it. And they'll probably get shocked or something and want to do something foolish. Also, you know, they might find out through a friend. Like a friend might say, "Oh well, this happened to me and that happened." And it's like, they'll say, "The same thing's happening to you, just the way it happened to me." And the person just get scared, you know. And a lot of times, they'll get misinformed. There's always a way of finding out.

It's sort of scary, even though I don't like to admit it to nobody. It's real scary. The fact that you know that you could be on this a long time. It's just scary because you know what you got is real serious. They tell you it's serious, it's not a joke. It's scary to know that you got something so strong and powerful inside you, and you just really wonder, "Am I gonna make it?" That's the negative times.

When they told me, and before I got the treatment, I was like, "Wow, I got cancer." I never thought that it would happen to me, and at first I thought it would be great because I'd be getting a lot of attention from everybody. But then when I started getting the treatment I saw how sick I got. One morning I woke up and I noticed that I was losing my hair, and then I got crazy, and I started asking myself, "Why me? Why did this happen to me?" Like a lot of times I just feel so angry 'cause, "Why couldn't it be somebody else? Why has this happened to me?" I thought, "There's all these guys doing wrong, killing people, dealing drugs, why couldn't it have been somebody like that and instead it was me, and I wasn't doing nothing wrong." At first the thought did cross my mind, "Did I do something wrong when I was younger?" and I asked the doctor and he said, "It's nothing that you did in the past, that you was a bad boy or anything. Don't worry it's nothing that you committed a sin or anything that you did in the past. It happens. It just comes up."

I have plenty of strange dreams. A lot of times, I'd dream, like I'd feel like I'm falling. And you know I'm just like folding over a little. And I feel like I'm falling, I would jump, you know, and pull myself together. And I'd wake up, I'd be in the middle of the bed. It was kind of strange. I feel like I'm just, like, rolling over sometimes. The last time I felt like I was going off a cliff. I was just laying on the edge of the cliff, and I felt like I was rolling off, and I jumped, tried to hang on to the edge of the cliff. Once I hit the bottom, but it was, like, the only thing I saw was, I saw myself, you know, I felt like I was watching myself, right, I was like looking from another spot. And I saw myself going like this and, like, when I was about to hit the floor everything went blank and all I saw was a bunch of little stars. And then I would wake up. I haven't had that dream in a long time.

Sometimes I have nightmares. Like, I remember when I first

came here, you know, I was really scared, 'cause one night I woke up screaming and I was in a cold sweat. 'Cause I dreamed that I was right there by the nurses' station, and this was like after it was, like, around one o'clock at night, in the morning. And it's like there was nobody around, 'cause there's like two or three nurses running on the floor and they was all busy, and there was nobody there. And I remember, I was, I went to the nurses' station to get something and nobody was there, so I had a remote control car. So I was just there, just waiting to see who would come. And nobody came, so I started driving around my little remote control car. Then I dreamed that I went to the edge, you know, to the corner of the nurses' station, right, and it's like, I drove it way down the hall. It's like I was trying to get the car to come back, and the car kept going and then it turned. And you know, I was like, trying to make the car come back, and it wouldn't come back. So I went after the car, went to get it, and then it's funny, 'cause I went around the corner, I saw the car, it was like, smashed to bits. And then it's like, some tall man, you know, I didn't even see his face, all I saw was a big huge body, with an axe. And I saw the guy sever my head and I woke up screaming that night. You know, I was like, I was really scared. The thing, it looked so real, it was so real. And I woke up screaming 'cause one of the parents told me. I remember I was in the four bedroom, and one of the parents told me that I woke up screaming, so she ran and got the nurse. And I woke up and the nurse was there and I was scared and jumping, the whole thing, I didn't want to go to sleep.

That was, like, the first time I had a nightmare of the hospital. And for some time I was scared to go past that corner after those hours 'cause, 'cause I remember one time, that I was here, I was up in the nurses' station, and it looked, everything looked exactly like in the dream. And I was really scared. I was looking around like, "Whoa, this is scary!" The only thing that was missing was the little remote control car. And it was scary, but I walked around the corner just so I could lose my fear. Everything was alright, so, that's how I lost the fear of it.

You got to look at the good side of it because out of every bad thing something good comes out of it. What came good out of this sickness was I met my girlfriend because a friend of mine in the hospital that was sick was her cousin and I went to my friend's house and stayed over a weekend and that's when I met her, and she's been very helpful to me. She's the only person that I'm really close to and she's the only one that I really talk to and I'm sort of glad that I have her because with her she makes it a little bit easier. Up to a point, I was keeping it in, then I met my girlfriend. Like times when I'm down and depressed, she always talks to me, and she tells me if I ever need someone to talk, to talk to her and every time I feel bad or something, she talks to me and I talk to her, and it feels better when you let it out. And it's like, sometimes I tell her that there's stuff that's really depressing me, sometimes. And even though you know, I mean it looks like I'm a happy guy, but a lot of times I just use that as a front to really hide the way I feel. And I would just tell her, like, that this stuff is horrible. I hate it, but I'll still do it, you know, as long as I know that in the future, I will be able to enjoy my life and, you know, without having to really think about it. And I speak to her about that kind of stuff.

Sometimes these two nurses, they just listen to me. The greatest thing is that they just listen. They listen, and you know, once in a while, they'll tell me something to make me feel better. You know, something to keep me going, to encourage me, like, they would tell me, well like sometimes I'm like tired of this, and it's been two years and I'm getting tired of it. And they're like, well, just, they'll tell me to think about the things that I'd like to fight for, that I'm really fighting this cancer for. And they would tell me, "Think about the future, what would you like to see?" how things are gonna be when, you know, in the future time. And mostly the reason why I fight the most is for that and for my girlfriend 'cause she cares for me. And I asked her once or twice, you know, "What would you do if I would die or something?" And the first time I asked her she started to cry, and said, "Don't talk about that 'cause I couldn't deal with it, or something." And that's mainly the reason why I fight so much. And the other reason is 'cause I'm a fighter, I just don't give up.

At first, when I first got sick, and they told me my hair was gonna fall out, I was like, "Oh God," that's it. 'Cause you know, before I got sick I was like, you know, like—not to sound all like that but, you know, a lot of girls liked me and all this, and I liked a lot of girls. And you know I was, like, friendly with everybody. And then when they told me my hair was going to fall out. I was, like, all the girls are gonna look at me and go, "Ee-oow, he's ugly, he's bald, and funny looking." And then I figured they'd be like, "Oh he got cancer, get away from him." And it scared me. I was like, that's it for my social life. I thought it was going to destroy it. But I was wrong. 'Cause like, I noticed now, I get just the same amount of girls as I had before. But I was really scared, 'cause I thought it was gonna prevent me from having friends. You know 'cause, I figured some people would be afraid 'cause they don't understand the disease, and they'll be afraid of socializing 'cause they don't really know and think they might catch it or something.

But, you know, with girls, well it's kinda of great though. 'cause it's like, we have, like for a guy, I say it's great 'cause we, we have, a very, a very small chance of getting a girl pregnant and all this. This is from what the doctors was telling me, 'cause I've asked them. You know, and it's like your chances are real small, you know, you could really, you know, get around to a girlfriend, you know, and not worry about it.

But then again, you have to use them 'cause you know, 'cause, you're, um, you have to use them though because you could catch an infection real easy. You know it's like, you have greater chances than anybody else of getting an infection. So it's like in a way it's good, and in a way it's not. 'Cause it's like, and especially if a guy, you know, he's like, he sleeps around, and he has a lot of girlfriends, you know, it's really wise to use a condom because it's like, from one girl to another girl, it's like, something could develop from that.

When I first found out about the cancer, I really didn't think about getting it on, 'cause I really didn't have that on my mind. But then, after a while, I started thinking, "Will this effect me, having children in the future?" or, "Will I be able to do that?" And then I started asking questions like, um, well, what will happen, and what are the chances of me having children and all this. And I even asked the doctor, you know, like, what are the chances of—suppose I had a child, and what are the chances of that child having cancer. And the doctor told me that the chances are, as if, the chances that my children have it are the chances that your children have it. Meaning that, it won't matter if I have cancer or not, so, if they get it, it's like, it's out of pure chance. So it's nothing really to worry about. And it really doesn't affect, you know, like, it doesn't affect the way you get aroused, or, when you get in the mood for it, it won't affect it. It's like, you'll be the same. There's really no difference, it's just that your sperm changes. That's about it.

You just gotta take your treatment and keep the faith, that's the way my mother puts it. You pray to God. You pray that everything will be alright. I got my whole family praying for me. When you feel sick and just feel bummed out, just think of the bright side. I always thought that, a whole year of this, I thought I would miss a whole year out of my life, but then I would think, "Yo, it's better to do this now than to do it later.

I'll get it over with now, and then I'll have the rest of my life to live."

I think, out of all people, your family are the people that get affected the worst. Like, the family is scared for you. Like, mostly the parents. It's like the parents see you suffering and though you know they'll feel bad 'cause it's like, the parents will be like, well that's a child of mine and he's suffering. And parents just can't see that. They can't see a child of their own suffering because of a disease or something. It's like it really hurts them, you know, to see them suffering and all that. It's like they go through the sickness with you 'cause they're always there, pushing you and helping you through. And they're like, they keep you going but, you know, it really affects them a lot because they see the way it affects you and the way you feel about it and how you get, and the way your attitude changes toward things.

The first time I had cancer, my mother was sad and she cried a lot, and that made me feel bad to see my mother crying because of my sickness. I wished that there was something I could do to help her, and she would just tell me, "Let me cry." But then the second time, when it relapsed, because my mother had plans for taking me and moving to Puerto Rico. So when it came back, my mother was angry. She was angry because it was always her dream to take the family to Puerto Rico. She was also angry that it came back, that I had to go through all that suffering again, not to mention that she would suffer with it too because of all those sleepless nights worrying about me and all this, and her being in the hospital with me, and it was real tough for my mother.

I think she's had it worse than I have because the way I started out was a lot different to the way I am now. I was different, I was like, I wasn't thinking back then the way I'm thinking now. I face the facts. I know my disease is very powerful and I know nobody really knows about it and that they

really don't know if I might go or not, but I ain't living negative or nothing, I just feel as though I should enjoy myself as
much as I can 'cause you never know. I wasn't like that before.
I used to take everything one step at a time, and now it's like I
rush things. Like if I want to do something, like there would
be a party and she would say, "Not this weekend. I want you
home this weekend. Save it for next weekend." And I would
say, "What the heck, I got my whole life." But now it's like,
not that I feel I'm gonna die, but I'm just having as much fun
as I can because if I ever do go, I did enjoy myself. My mother
is giving me more liberty now 'cause she knows I'm sick and
she understands me. So it's like I go out more. I go dancing, I
go to parties, I go out with my friends, and she understands
that.

At times, we did have our little quarrels because I was sick
and my mother had it all inside, and that's the way she would
get it out. My mother, she's a very proud person. She's not the
type to come out and talk it out. Instead, she would show me
in another way. Like she used to show me that she was worried and all that, and she used to yell at me, and talk about my
sickness, you know a problem to the family and all this. But I
would understand that 'cause I knew the way my mother
was, that she wasn't the type to tell me that she was worried.
But when she would come out like this, I would understand
her. She used to yell at me, and I'd just take it. Sometimes
when she would yell at me, I'd just tell her that I'd love her,
and I would hug her, and I knew that would make her feel a
lot better. A lot of times we had a lot of quarrels because of my
sickness. Sometimes she would sound like it was my fault that
I was sick, and I would tell her it's not really my fault. But
sometimes I lose my nerve when she tells me that, "You're
sick and you're ruining me."

Before I got sick my mother and my father were together,
and then they got divorced, and she made it sound like they

got divorced because of my sickness. I know myself it was not like that 'cause even before I got sick I noticed that they were falling apart, that they were going their ways. Then my father, he left for Colombia. He knew I was sick. He was there for me when I needed him, but then he started his life over. He said he's gonna come back for me so don't think he's abandoned me. Sometimes my mother makes it seem like he just left because of my sickness, and sometimes that would be the basis of the argument.

And you know, and I saw, I noted that it really affected my father a lot. And I think, in a lot of ways, that's why he left for Columbia. Because it really got to him, because I remember once my father, you know, he wasn't the kind of guy to let anybody see his tears come down. But I caught him a few times crying over the fact that I'm sick. 'Cause I remember once that I was, like, all hooked up to a lot of IVs and it's like, you know, I was really sick and I was sleeping. And I was like half and half, half awake and half asleep, and I remember waking up and I was like in a daze. Right, and I see my father sitting there in a chair just with his head down, crying, you know, quietly. I knew he was crying 'cause he looked up and I saw him wipe his tears. And I just, I like, I went back out again. I went back to sleep. I felt really bad and I was, like, I wanted to tell him, "Don't cry for me 'cause it's not as bad as it looks." 'Cause like nothing came out.

When you think about it, it's like, it really makes you feel all sentimental and stuff 'cause you know, even though a lot of times, you know, like, your father, like, my father, you know 'cause when I was small I used to get into a lot of trouble, and he used to punish me and all this. And I used to, like, oh, he doesn't love me 'cause he punished me and he spanks me once in a while. But then, when I saw that, I thought, you know, 'cause, when, at the moment that my father punished me and he spanks me or whatever, I think oh, that I hate him and all this. But when I saw him that day, I saw him crying, I was like, you know, yeah, he punished me and all this, but he does it 'cause he loves me.

When my brother found out, he didn't know about it 'cause that was a time that we was having, like, family problems and he, my brother, didn't come around for a while. When he got married and there was all these problems. So one time he came over to the house to see my mother and to see me. I was still in stitches, and he noticed that patches of my hair was falling out, and then my mother told him that I got cancer, and then my brother started to cry, and says, "Why you?" He felt real bad, and he hugged me and all this, and he's just telling me, "Don't worry about it, it's gonna be alright." And ever since then, he would come around. It makes us closer. Now my brother, what my mother and my brother had against each other, it's like it's over with, and my brother comes regularly, he comes whenever he could. In a way, this is another good thing that the sickness brought.

And you know, he'd be real nice to me that I, well, that I got to keep fighting, and we're gonna do this, and we're gonna do that when you get older. It's like just keep your mind on it, when you get older we're gonna be driving around in cars and we're gonna be together, and have a good time. And you know, he really encourages me, he's like, like protective of me. I remember once, somebody made a remark about my sickness. And they said something really dumb, that was really low. But I really didn't let it get to me, but, you know, my brother heard this, and he got real angry. He's like, well, that's not something that you should talk about that way, 'cause just think, suppose you have it, or God forbid, what if one of your children have it, you know, you wouldn't think of it that way. Because it's like it could happen to anybody. It's like my brother told him that disease, it don't matter if you're black or white or what your religion is, or whatever. It doesn't discriminate you. It's like, anybody could get sick and it could happen to anybody. It's like, it's not really funny. You know, it's not something to make fun about. And it's like my brother told him, you know, I understand if you don't know about it, but it's like, you shouldn't talk about it like that either.

It's good when you have friends and you meet other people your age who have the sickness. Every time I meet somebody I'm real friendly with them, and when I find out they got my sickness, I understand. I met this guy here and I got to know him and I'm like, "Yo, you know I know how it is because I have the same thing." You know we understand each other, you know how it is. When I first met him, he used to tell me, "Yo, don't worry about it, everything's gonna be alright." I used to tell him the same, and we used to, like, encourage each other, and we used to be together a lot, and that's how we are now, we're always together.

There are some people who just close themselves in like a shell and don't let nobody in. I don't advise that 'cause when you do that it gets to you. 'Cause I know a few friends of mine like that and they have died and I think it's because they never opened up to anyone, they never really talked about what they felt. There's always someone who's going to be there to talk to you, there's always people that take a liking to you and they want to be there for you. All I can say for other people is like, open up to other people when there's some-body that offers you a chance to be there. I could understand that the person would be depressed, but eventually just try to open up.

I wasn't the person to open up, I wasn't like that, at first I was all to myself, but then I noticed that I needed to talk to people. Like for me, I have a good friendship with two nurses. I consider them like my sisters, and they consider me like their little brother they never had. They always talk to me and I talk to them. I learned this from a friend that I met when I first started. They amputated his leg, but he got a prosthesis, and he's great now. He comes to see me now and then, and I go to his house and stay over. We're good friends, but when he was sick, this guy was real cool, and I sort of like picked up from him. I used to see the way he was, he was like my role model. He was always smiling, he always had a good laugh, always had a joke, he was friendly with everyone. When he met me, he told me that the sickness is a real bummer, but, "Yo, don't worry about it, you could still have a lot of fun with your sickness and all." I'm friendly with everybody 'cause I got that from him. I learned to live with my sickness and I learned it from him 'cause I saw the way he was. Now that he's cured he says, "Yo, don't worry about it 'cause you're going to be cured too. Look at me." And you know, he comes and visits.

I like to do art, what is called graffiti, but I don't do it on the walls, I do it on paper. When I draw, I draw the way I feel, like when I feel a certain way that's the way I'm gonna draw. I met this guy, Gary, God rest his soul, and we really understood each other because he was from the same parts I was from. We understood each other 'cause we spoke the same language, he was a graffiti artist too. And when he died, the nurses were afraid to tell me because they knew that I was close to this guy. I considered him like my brother, and I would talk to him, and we talk about the same things. When the nurses told me that he died, I was shocked 'cause I remember the way I saw him the last time and he looked so good, he looked healthy like there was nothing wrong with him. We were on different cycles, getting our chemo at different times. I came in and when I was leaving he would come in like two days before I left and the last time I was gonna see him he wasn't there. So I was like, "Where's Gary?"

Then the nurses were afraid to tell me, they would avoid it. I would ask them something about Gary and the nurses would change the subject. At first I didn't realize and they would say, "He's feeling real sick. I don't think you should go see him." And then I started to realize, wait a minute, there's something funny here, 'cause then I went to the board and I didn't see his name on it and I said, "What's going on here?" That's when one of the nurses pulled me over and she took me to my room to sit down, and she broke it to me real nice.

All that day, the nurses were so nice. They were talking to me, and asking me, how I was and they was being there for me. They knew how I felt because me and Gary, we felt like brothers and they knew that I would have a bad reaction. I was surprised, then I felt so bad. I was like, "Man, Gary, he was cool." And in a way, I felt disappointed because that was somebody for me. I thought that Gary was put there for me, and I felt like he was taken away from me. I felt bad and depressed because he was like a brother to me, and I still keep thinking that he's my brother and he's still around for me. I started thinking that if Gary died and he was all healthy and he was well-built and muscular, I figured that I'm going into that same fate, and I felt real bad. I felt depressed for a while, and then eventually, like they say in my neighborhood, I woke up and smelled the coffee, because I got out of the trance, I was like in a trance, even though to the nurses, I would play it off like there was nothing wrong. But when I would be in my room by myself, I would realize how much I missed this guy.

One day I asked for some things. I asked for a picture of Gary, and I asked for the dates, the day he was born and the day he died, he died on Valentine's Day. That was a real bummer, in a way. I was thinking how his girlfriend felt because he was close to his girlfriend, and the way I heard it she came on Valentines Day, and she found out. That must have hurt to lose your valentine on Valentine's Day, out of all days, and I could imagine how she must have felt. So I got all this background on him, and I just started drawing, and I put, "We'll be chillin"—that means we'll be together, we'll be alright, we'll always be together—I put, "We'll be chillin" and I put it real nice, and I drew a character of him, and then I drew this on a big piece of cardboard paper, and then I took construction paper and I stapled the cardboard on the construction paper, and on the construction paper, I put his picture, and underneath his picture, I put the card from his funeral, the wake, and underneath I put the day he lived and the day he died. I put together all these things, and all around it I wrote poems, like, "God rest his soul, wherever you're at, you may be happy," and I put like little sayings, "Peace my brother, that you'll always be with me, I'll always remember you." And I started putting the names of his friends and my friends that we knew each other.

It was a big project, and I just did it. Nobody asked me to. As an artist, I thought like when artists know each other and something happens to one, it's like they all pay tribute to him, so I did that nice piece for him. And back home, we did like this project. We went to this park, and my cousin talked to some people and we got permission to do a piece on the handball court and we did this nice piece, my cousin did this for me because he knew the way I felt for Gary, and people respected it. They didn't deface it, and it was up there for months and months.

You have to just think positive. And it's like, you know, everything, it's like, take your treatment 'cause it'll work for your benefit. 'Cause at the moment you'll be like, "Oh these people are just torturing me," but then afterwards, after you're done, you're like, "Oh, I'm really glad that I went through all of it 'cause like now, I could live my life and be happy." And now I'm like, I understand it. They should just, don't let it sink you down. You know, don't let it bring you down and just keep a positive attitude. That's the way I see it.

Even though, you know, at times it's really hard to really keep your hopes up. Like when you get sick you're like, you know, this stuff is terrible. I don't see what good it's doing, it's like it's doing more harm than good. And it's like, just go through those times, just bear with it 'cause the other times is going to be, you know, better. It's like, I'm really glad, 'cause, it's like, I have this sickness and a lot of good came, you know, 'cause with the bad, there's also good that comes with it. And I made a lot of friends. And I've got to do a lot of things that I've never done before. And it's like, you know, in a lot of ways, it's like, this has like improved the way I am. It's like now I'm more understanding.

You know, 'cause I used to make fun of people, other people that were sick and all this. And it's like now I understand how it feels, and now I don't think of it as kind of funny. It's not really funny at all. And it's like, now, in a way, not that I'm glad that I got sick, but it's like now I understand it more. It's like, when I hear about someone else, I could be more understanding to the person. And this way, I feel I talk to them and help them out. I'm more considerate of other people with other diseases. Like, I'm more understanding. 'Cause before, it's like, I'd be like, well, they've got diseases, and these people are weird, and you know, I want to stay away from them. It's like now, I'm more open-minded. It's like, I'm willing to talk to the person and it could be any disease, it won't bother me. I'll just, you know, talk to the person and I won't act differently. Back then, I would act, you know, I would act like, keep your distance, and all this. But now I'm like, I'll be closer to the person. And I really won't treat 'em that way, like, keep your distance and make fun of the person. This disease has opened my mind to a lot of things. Now I'm more understanding of anything. Like if someone would tell me something about a problem or something, I'll be more open-minded and try to help the person out. 'Cause ever since I got sick I'm trying to help everybody out with their sickness and stuff, and keep them going. That way I keep going.

Just keep an open mind to everything. That's the way I see it now. I just keep an open mind. And don't let it get to you. 'Cause it's like, some people that start thinking, "Oh, the best way is to kill myself, that's the best way out." That's garbage. At one point I had thought about it myself. Like, the second time I got sick I was, you know, thinking that I'm sick and tired of this disease 'cause every time I want to do something, the sickness, it gets in the way. And you can't do this thing, you have to like work around it. And I was like, I'm tired of it. And you know, just, I said the best way out is if I take my life and I won't have to go through this. But then you know, some, a few friends of mine spoke to me, it was like, that's not the way out. 'Cause it's like, don't think it's gonna do this, just end it. And you know, you're gonna keep, you're gonna be wondering if I would have stayed alive would I have made it. You know, you're gonna be wondering for eternity, could I have done it.

And you know, not only for yourself, but it's like, you gotta think about others. Like how it's gonna affect other people if you kill yourself. Like, my, my friend that spoke to me, 'cause you know, a lot of people thought that I was going to commit suicide. At times I was thinking about it. When I got sick again, a lot of people noticed that I was depressed a lot. And it's like, I wasn't as cheery as I used to be. This was for a while, and at that time, well, my friends talked to me. They said, "Well, just think about it and think about how it's going to affect your parents." My friends spoke to me, they like, they talked me out of it. And my mother was like, "Well I love you a lot," you know, and "It will really hurt me, a lot. A lot more if you did that than just enduring and just, get it over with."

At that time, there was like, very few people that I could say it to. I was like, at first I really didn't tell anybody what my thoughts were. You know, and then people started noticing, 'cause like here on the floor it's like noticeable, it's like, it's been so long the nurses get to know how you are and know your feelings. They just get to know you and just be able to know these things. And it's like, you know, people started noticing that I was like slowing down, like winding out. It was like something's going on, and they spoke to people that were close to me, to talk to me, and try to get me to talk and get it out of me. They told Arturo and Arturo spoke to me and we talked then, I talked to my mother, and then my girlfriend spoke to me. It's very important to have some people to talk to, 'cause if you don't, you know, all of that is going to be in you and it's gonna pile on. And it don't matter how strong a person is, but there's always gonna be a point where it's gonna build up and a person is either gonna have to talk or they, or the low is gonna affect them.

It's like it shouldn't be hard to talk to someone you know. I mean, it's always easier to speak to someone that had the sickness or has it, and that person understands you, but it's also good to speak to other people you know. That way they could at least get a chance to understand you. The way I see it, it's always good to give everybody a chance to explain their sickness and how you feel about it and then in the future that person is not going to be the same as the person who had the sickness. And they'll be able to help you out. And that's the most important thing, to be able to talk about it. Like, you don't have to speak to everybody, but just to have one or two people that you could level with, and that you're open with and you could just come straight out and tell them how you feel.

And not worry about telling them. 'Cause there's like, certain people, this happens to me, you know that you feel insecure and you don't want to talk to them because of some reason. You're just afraid of telling them 'cause the person might, you really don't know how the person is going to react. You might be afraid that if you talk to this person like that, if you're open with them, that they'll just run away from you, or they'll back up. But there's always other people that, like with me, my nurse, right? We started talking and it's, like, I instantly felt like I could confide in her, I could trust her with the way I felt, and not worry about her. You know, like doing anything drastic like, 'cause I was thinking, you know, I was worrying, at first I was like, if I tell her will she tell anyone else? You know, not really that I didn't want her to tell anybody, but I just didn't want the whole world to know about it. You know and I was like, at first I was scared. But then, I just took that chance and said, "Hey, what the heck." I told her the way I felt, that once in a while it got to me and I got depressed once in a while, and I was scared. Like for some reason you just don't want everybody to know the way you really felt. I really don't like everybody to know the way I am.

The best thing is to have a friend to speak to. It helped me a lot. And the best part is, that you know, I'm friendly with just about everybody. So that's like the best part. Try, even though at times the chemo will make you grouchy, you may not want to talk to anybody. But you just try, you know, make an effort, to speak to people and be friendly as much as you can. Like a lot of people, that worked with me, they helped me through my sickness, right, they understand the way it is, they already know how the chemo reacts. Like, 'cause like with a friend of mine I told, "Be a trooper, just don't let it get to you, just be a trooper." That's the way I see it.

And you know, like a lot of times, some people don't understand and you really can't push it that much. Like 'cause, like when my friend was getting sick, it's like I noticed that her mother was like, "Will you cut it out already? You don't have to do this." And I told her, you know, you don't understand.

Because it's not that you want to do this, it just happens. My friend was throwing up a lot. She was really sick. And it's like, a lot of times you can't really fight it but, in your mind you just, you keep fighting it. You just don't put your guard down, you know? But it's like you really can't push it because some people don't understand and think that you're just, that you're just acting it up. Like some people will get depressed and get really grouchy and don't want to speak to anyone and the other person that doesn't understand would, they'll misinterpret it. 'Cause they'll think that you're just being, you know, you're just being mad at the world. But a lot of times, the other person don't understand. Just try to understand and not speak too much 'cause a lot of times when a person is getting chemo they really don't want to hear it. And you know they'll just come off grouchy and a lot of times, this has happened to me.

I had, like, my mother would tell me something and I'll just snap at her, and tell her something that I really don't mean. And at the moment it's just because I'm just grouchy because of chemo, and it really gets to me sometimes. I get angry and then when there's somebody telling me something that I don't want to hear, you know, you just snap at it, you just go all out. And even when it's like for people who really don't understand it, you know, that really don't know how it is, just try to be understanding. Like don't push it too much. It's good to be encouraging but there's a point that you can't go over because then it's going to be like, pushing and then the person is going to be like, "Hey, don't push me."

'Cause that's how it was with my friend. Her mother was telling her, "Why are you such a grouch?" and all this, and my friend just told her, "It's just, 'cause I feel like it, and just stay out of my life, 'cause I didn't ask you." And I just told the mother, I said, "Don't mind it, it's not, it's that because of the chemo she's coming out like that, so she really doesn't feel good and then you try to push it, 'cause you're pushing a little too much. Then she's not going to appreciate it." And I told her mother, "Just, don't really pay no mind to what she's saying 'cause she really doesn't mean it. It's just that she doesn't feel good right now. She'll just snap at anybody because of the pain that she's feeling, you know?"

That happens to everyone I speak with—my friends and, you know, especially with me, 'cause at times I could be real patient but at other times I have a short temper. And it's like, people are liable to say things that they really don't mean. And they'll just snap and say things because they're feeling pain inside. And it's like, you know, if there's somebody else on the outside trying to help him out but the person on the outside doesn't really know how to help out, and they'll say something, they'll say something and the person, they'll just take it another way and they'll think it's like, "Oh well, you don't know about this and you never felt this way before, so you're just saying that 'cause you don't know about it. But if you knew you wouldn't be saying that." That happens a lot, and it affects everybody in a way, even in the smallest way, 'cause once in a while, someone'll say something and then a patient, the person with cancer, will, they'll catch an attitude or they'll take it wrong. They'll take it differently. 'cause a person might say something and mean it in a certain way, but the patient wouldn't take it in that way, they'll take it in another way.

People should like, they should be ready for a change in the attitude. Before a sickness, the patient might be easygoing, calm, and all that. But then during the, um, getting the treatment, like, and the person will be, like, they'll be grouchy, and they'll be a totally different person. You know it's like, the people around the patient should, like, try to be understanding, just have an open mind 'cause you know, it'll happen, just be expecting it. Don't be expecting it but, it's like, when it happens, just don't take it the wrong way, just don't really pay no mind, just try to talk it out. Like after the person finishes the chemo, the cycle, it's up to the person. 'Cause I say that's the reason why, at least with me, that's the reason why I snap out sometimes, at my mother, or other people that tell me something and they really don't know how it is. And you know I'll tell them, I'll just tell them off. But I just know it's because of the pain I'm feeling inside and there's somebody trying to help you but they don't know how to help so it's like, you like, you try to pull away from the person. And the best way to pull away is by telling them something that you know will make the person just back off. 'Cause that's like the biggest thing. Like with the attitude changes.

You know the people around them should be understanding, and try to be a little helpful. 'Cause a lot of times, instead of just saying something, and trying to push, it'll help a lot more if you just be a buddy like, be there. You know, just stand there and you really don't have to say anything just as long as, just your presence will help a lot. Just being there.

Just think about the good days

They told me that I had a tumor in my leg, and it was like a huge tumor, really big, and they did like surgery to find out if it was malignant. When the doctor came in, he told me that it was malignant. Back then I thought that it was not cancerous, I misunderstood it. I thought malignant meant reversal, no cancer, and nonmalignant means you have cancer, so it wasn't no shock then, so when he told me, I was happy. Until, like, he kept on talking to my father, and then talking like that, and that's when, when I first found out I had it. From there on that's when they started treatment, and he told me I had to go to the hospital for two months to get treatment so that my tumor would shrink down, so that they could do an operation and take it all out at one shot. That's when I came here.

At first, when you come to treatment, I wouldn't want my worst enemy to have that, throwing up when you get nauseous, seeing orange stuff coming out of your stomach and you haven't eaten nothing, and green stuff coming out and you haven't eaten nothing. It's really sick and you get a raw taste in your mouth. I wouldn't want nobody to go through that and especially the pain that I went through. I wouldn't want nobody to go through that. I see other patients here, we had a group and we used to play poker, and that's when they told me everything that would be happening about chemotherapy. It's not nice.

They tell you these things but you're not shocked or you're not scared, you're not like, "Hey the doctor said you've got a 50–50 chance," and you're not scared, and then you go through the treatment and you're like I can't wait 'til next year comes and then one month, and it's a whole year, and everything is done, so you're finally cured, so you're like, "Hey man, I can have a party and celebrate." But when it's the time when it comes back and you have to do it again, that's when the depression starts, because when you get hit by it the first time you don't know what you're in for, but when you get hit by it the second time, that's what happened to me. It hit me on my back, close to my lungs or my ribs next to my spine, and then that's when I started to get pain. He wanted to kill it, he wanted to shrink it down, as close as possible, and that's when the depression starts. I guess it really blew me away. That's when they were saying they would probably bring a psychiatrist up to talk to me.

I never came myself to say that I was really depressed, you know like, "Hey you gonna die." That's the worst fear because what really scared me was, I'm not no fool, I've been here a year and a half going on two years, and there have been patients here, and when they go on that scan, when they stick you to see how your heart rate is, that was scary because that's when they are checking to see how your heart is, and any time it goes in your lung, nine out of ten, you can pack it up. Because Paul passed away, Graciella passed away with a brain tumor in her head, and David passed away, and it's frightening, it's really frightening, to find out all your friends that you've been playing with and partying with are going. You know all that's going to happen, and the first time, you're scared or whatever, but when it comes back the second time you're really frightened, and that's the scariest part of it.

You know, after when it's in remission, you're like, "Hey it's all over," but then it comes back to do everything it did all over again, throwing up, nausea, it's ridiculous. And then to know that they said you had a good time, passing it off, getting into remission, and then it comes back, and you may not make it again. 'Cause I know Graciella, she passed away but she'd been sick seven years, in and out, seven years back and forth. But those kids had more complications than I had, like in the lungs, a couple were in the lungs, one or two were in the brain, a lot had passed away, and it frightened me that they did pass away. I don't know how to put it, you would say one of those tough luck, passing away which you don't want it to happen. When the doctors will not tell you, all they will tell you is he passed away from the cancer, they will not tell you the complications and everything, which they are not allowed to, but I still find out, you hear people talking, or whatever.

Like once I had a friend she was sick in the hospital, she didn't have cancer, but she overheard somebody talking about her best friend in the hospital who had cancer, and she overheard, and they said there's nothing else we can do about it. That's when she got really depressed, and she let it out on me, so I got to know, like to find out that the doctors cannot do nothing else because there are so many complications where it had came into the tumor, in the head, and in the lungs, and all over, where it's out of their hands, where they can't do anything, and she was telling me that, she was, it was so bad. You see how bad cancer can take over.

It's scary, you don't want it to happen, and other times you're like well I just hope it doesn't happen to me because in some patients the way they pass away so fast, you know some may not last long. By the time you get in here and start chemotherapy, it's already to an extent where it's only but so little they can do. If you catch it in the beginning it's more better, the chance, but this other guy I know, he had the same thing I had, and this was after I had the operation, he had talked to my mother and he was thinking he could have the same operation done as I had. But his, by the time he came in, was so huge, they couldn't do anything, and they had to amputate, and then he had a lot of complications, both lungs was full of tumors, and he had just come out of having an operation with just one side done, and they didn't know when they could complete the other side. That's really scary to know that it's going, that's when they told me that it had came back.

If they would have told me that it was in the lungs I probably would have had mobile depression. How they say, mobile depression, when you're really sick and depressed. I don't know what they call it, but in my terms, when a person's real real depressed. If they had told me that, with all that I know, with all the patients passing away, and the majority of them had it in the lung and that's when they stopped breathing. It doesn't take any longer to put two and two together. I've been here two years, it ain't like I don't know anything and I'm not hearing anything.

What happened was when they told me it came back, they made a mistake of putting the EKG on me, that's to monitor your heart, and I had seen all my friends with it in the lungs before they passed away with EKGs on them, and that like frightened me real real bad. I thought I was going. So a nurse came in and was talking to me and found out that that's what I was really scared about so she took 'em off. I know that with most of the patients that passed away, the last thing they do is monitor your heart, knowing that I'm going to pass away, but the doctors didn't tell me that. It was very frightening and scary. What happened was they had the chemotherapy too strong that he had gave me. That's when I had real severe pains in the chest, and that's when they had the EKGs on me, and it was hard to breath. Then a couple days later, the doctor came in and I just confronted him, and I said, "Am I gonna die or what?" and he said, "You'll be the first to know if you're going to." And that relieved me when they took off the EKGs.

But I had so much pain before then, where I couldn't lay down, couldn't sit up, I was taking Percocet and Percocet wasn't helping, and they were going to give me morphine, but I didn't know morphine came in a pill, I thought it came in a shot, and I was frightened of shots, so that's why I didn't take it, but it was so awkward with the pain that I guessed that the tumors were in the lungs. That was for about four days, I was frightened for four days. I was praying, which anybody else would do. Like you're thinking that the world is going to end, and you hope that you're going to heaven. You hear so much about the promised lands and all that, so you're hoping that you're going there, but then you sinned so much, and it's like that's when you're like moaning to yourself because I know I'm gonna die, but I didn't die yet, and it's like really hectic.

A couple of the nurses came in and I talked to one or two, and that's when it got back to the doctor, that's when they took off the EKGs. But before that, I remember a part when he came in, a nurse, and I was in so much pain, and he saw that I was in a lot of pain, and he bent down and said try to lay down and see if that will help, and the pain was so bad, he saw me, I guess my eyes were rolling, and I was in so much pain, he grabbed me, and when he grabbed me, I took in air but I couldn't let it out, and then he had lift me up so fast, he kept on lifting me up more, it finally came out, and that's when I yelled out in pain, it's like a lot of tears, it was really really severe, a lot of severe pain from the chest area. From what I understand now the chemotherapy that he gave me was much too strong for my body, because I only was like 120 pounds, and I couldn't take it.

That's one part of my life I don't want to remember. To

know that that was going to happen, to know what I know now, that it wasn't going to happen, but back then I was like scared out of my wits. It's like those days are so hard to remember because most of it, I was in tears and crying with the pain. My mother would bring me soup and food, and I couldn't eat none of it, and I was losing a lot of weight, and it was just like you would say set there to die because I wasn't eating much, it was hard to eat, every time you sit up it's pain, every time you lay down it's pain, and with the bed moving up and down every time it hits a position it's more pain, less pain, you can't get in the right position. All you could see from my face is shedding a lot of tears, a lot of tears.

My mother always would say, say the twenty-three psalms, and some other scriptures in the Bible, to repeat the psalms. It kind of comforts you a lot, but some other times the pain is so severe that it's pretty difficult. But I always wanted to live, I didn't want to go. Where you would hear other cases where they would want to die but not me, I wanted to live for everything I got.

I wouldn't want nobody to go through that and it's really, for the four days I'd been in pain, I just would hope that if it happens to another person, that if he feels comfortable praying, do that, or whatever he feels comfortable doing. Do it those four days while it's flashing through your mind that you're going to pass away and try to remember the good days that you had, and don't remember the bad days 'cause the bad days will get you depressed and the good days will kind of get you through it. Like if your parents took you on vacations, or if you ever went and saw a good movie, or you ever went ice skating, bike riding, or when you were small playing baseball, football, and just remember that, that will comfort you.

When you're in that pain, everything is flashing through your mind, and you don't want that to happen, because when that happens you're just about ready to give everything up, if

you're letting the pain get over you. Whereas I said before, I
always think a lot, I don't think about the bad days, I always
think about the good days, like now my mother is planning a
trip, we're going on a cruise, that will be nice. I'm looking
forward to that and to eating all that good food. Keep those
bad memories far apart from the good memories. If it ever
comes to the last day where you know you're gonna pass
away or don't have so long, just think about the good days.
But you have to go on with life. You just pray to God, and
hope it's not you next, and when it does happen you see all
the nurses crying and everything, and that's the day I
wouldn't like nobody to see. I can't picture myself in a coffin,
watching everybody mourn, I don't think I could live with
that. If I had my choice I'd die going to sleep, won't have
nothing to worry about.

So I've already gone through the worst so now I'm able to
cope with it. But in other cases, every time they hear it's come
back, it's like they feel like picking up something and throwing it on the floor. In my case, it's not like that. I guess I'm one
of the strong ones you'd say. A lot of the patients when they
come back they're not feeling well, they want to be alone, and
you would say, "I know it's bad, it's coming back, and you
have another year." I know it's a serious situation, but I don't
put it as a serious situation, whereas if it comes back, I'm not
putting a formula where you can die from cancer, unless you
get really sick, that's when it flashes back in my memory.
Other than that, I figure it out like cancer you cannot die from,
it's curable, that's how I live day by day, now that it's come
back. It's like a little more throwing up and regurgitating, and
hopefully, this same time next year I'll be done.

A lot of us say, "Why me?" but hey, they said cancer is in
everybody, it's in you, me, just depending if it forms up or
not. My mother had this apartment upstairs and she had
rented it to this guy and this guy told us, I don't know if he

called himself psychic or what, but I have a little handicapped brother, and he felt him and he said that he doesn't have cancer nowhere, and then he felt me and he said you have cancer in the leg, and I didn't tell him nothing, and he told me that I had it when I was about seven years old but it never formed up until now, and to know that all that time I've been going to the hospital and they never took x-rays or nothing like that, to know that it could have been cured back then, or if I had met him five years earlier, and he would have told me, "Go check out your leg," or something like that. I don't know if not to believe him or not, I don't know if I would have believed him, but I would have checked it out because it doesn't hurt.

When you hear the word cancer, that word is frightening, that's a word that stands out by itself. You tell somebody you got a tumor, "Oh, I hope it feels better." You tell them you got cancer, it's like it's the worst thing that happened, when you tell people that you have cancer, they're like sorry to hear that, it's like a depression to them. You know, that's why when I first started and I had cancer, I told everyone that I had cancer and I never liked the way they looked at me and tried to change the subject or try to look not depressed. That's why when they say, "What's the matter with your leg?" I say, "I broke it." I don't lie to them either because I did break my leg. I do have a tumor in my leg, so I'd tell people I have a tumor in my leg.

Everybody on my block knew when my leg got swollen up, I was back and forth to the hospital. They not seeing me around on the block, and they like, "Where's Joe? He's in the hospital." And I got a big brace on my leg that everybody could see, and I'm walking with crutches, so I was like, why lie, "I got cancer in my bone." And I really told everybody on my block so everybody knew my condition. And then they would like, "I'm sorry to hear that," and all depressed, like,

"You gonna die, man." And one stupid, crazy guy told me, "Oh man, if I had cancer, I'd rather them cut off my leg than give me a bone transplant." I looked at him as if he was stupid and said, "Yea, if you was in my place, you wouldn't be saying that, cut off my leg and I couldn't walk around with somebody else's leg," 'cause I really did have a bone transplant. So somebody tell you that, you just look at them like they're really stupid, because if it was you, you'd do everything the doctor says you can do. I didn't bother listening to him. But my real friends, they're OK. I go everywhere with them but I be on crutches so I go much slower. Some of them totally forgot that I'm sick, and they be like, "Yo, you want to go ice skating? Oh, I forgot you can't go ice skating."

My mother just told me recently that when she was small, when we were all small, she had a dream that she was pushing one of us in a wheelchair, and she didn't know who it was, and when my younger brother came handicapped, she thought it was him, and then he started walking so it wasn't him she was pushing in a wheelchair, and then my mother started to get mad at my older brother because I was her right-hand man and he never did nothing around the house. My brother, he doesn't want to be bothered. And my mother said, "After all these years, I finally see the one I was pushing in the wheelchair and that was you."

So, she's depressed because of all the kids, me, because I always be there. But nobody in the house is having thoughts that I'll pass away, and that reminds me, when I was in the hospital getting the operation, my mother would be there crying and crying and I'd be like, "Don't worry, Mom, nothing's gonna happen." My mother always cried for me because I never cried, and I don't like seeing her cry and that gets me real mad, so I will be pretty strong so that she won't cry, or if she does cry she doesn't cry around me, which I thank her for that because that would just make me mad. I want to be strong for her, strong for the rest of the family.

I always felt that—people say that—you have two types of patients, when it's an operation. There's a patient that's not worrying about the operation, and my mother is crying, and the operation will be like OK. "I'll go get the operation and I'll be back talking to you when I'm finished or I'll call you when I'm done." Then you have the other kid, "Oh, no, I don't want to take the operation, I'm scared," and all this, and I think that's worse on the parents, 'cause if the child is strong enough to face what he's having, then it's easier on the parents. When it's hard on the patient, than it's even harder on the parent because "I don't want my child having this, and you're hurting him."

If you're strong about something, like for instance this other girl, she doesn't like getting her IVs in her arm, and you hear her every night, and I think that's really depressing for the parents, but to find out if the patient is strong, the parents be like, "He's strong, and he'll pull through." Like, for me, hey, you have to get it done, so I'll get it done. Right now, if you were to speak with my mother she would say I have faith that he's gonna make it, like if I was weak or whatever, she'd probably be saying that but doesn't mean it, but my mother is saying it because she means it. If they go down and you're strong you'll be able to bring them back up. It's worse on your parents than it is on you because everytime they hear your name, they're crying. If you're eating and doing well, they're doing well, whereas if you're not doing well, they're like a depression.

I'm not looking on what's happening now, I'm looking on what's happening when I'm done and I don't have to come back to this stupid place to get no more chemotherapy, I don't have nothing to do with this hospital, I don't want to see no doctors, you know. I'll come back for a visit, you know, "How you doing, goodbye." You don't picture what's happening now, whatever has to be done, just get it done with, don't be bothered with it. Picture it this way, "I'm getting it done now, but a year from now, I'll be somewhere far gone, and I won't have to picture anything." What my mother does, since I've been sick, she'll try to plan something to take my mind off of it, like going on a cruise.

I used to have a few good friends and then when they found out, they never bothered, they never wanted to visit me. And then I had Dalton, he works with the helicopters over here, and he comes to visit me everyday, and I'm like, that's a true friend, and I said, "You're the best friend I ever had, and if I ever hit Lotto, don't worry, whatever I have, you have." A really true friend, you could say, I wouldn't have known this if I hadn't gotten sick. Now, I've been sick, he's been here, and if my mother can't come, he'll stop by my house, and say, "You want me to bring anything by Joe?"

In the beginning, the doctors they tell you what they think you know, they don't tell you what's really happening. You can find out all the information from them, and they'll tell you this and they'll tell you that, but if you're smart, you go to a patient that's going through this stuff and ask him. It's way different from what doctors tell you. Because they're the ones going through it. I was in that situation when I started out, but now that I've been here like a year and a half and I met this guy and he was just starting treatment, and they were telling him the different things that he can expect, nausea and all that, and I told him, "I'm not gonna lie to you, these are the things that are going to happen, you're not gonna like the medication, you're gonna start throwing up, you got some good things and some bad things that come out of it. For one thing, your hair falls off, all the hair on your body goes, and if you don't like being bald that's one thing you have to live

with, when it grows back it looks better than it did before."
My hair's not like this, not that curly, this is a good thing out
of chemotherapy.

And the other thing I be telling him is, "Your skin'll get all
ashy, and it'll start flaking, and sometimes you get sores in
your mouth, and sometimes there's something they get to
give you and you get pains in your stomach or whatever. The
doctors, they tell you, but I think you rather hear it from
somebody else that's been through the problems that you're
going through, 'cause you can always ask him something. If
you ask a nurse they'll be like, "I don't know, I never had
that," or they'll try to answer it as best as possible, but if you
ask a patient that's going through it then they can tell you the
difference, certain things you can do, like when you start in
treatment and you start throwing up. I suggest the best thing
that you can do is tell your mother to bring you soup because
you not gonna eat nothing else, like if you feel like you gonna
throw up, and it can't come up, it's so hard, drink a glass of
water, so when you throw up it will come liquid, or else you
feel like you're bringing up your insides."

I would tell him that, try to take it as best as possible, and I
would tell him everything that he's in for, what he should
expect. I would tell him, like the best food that you eat you
won't like it after awhile because of chemotherapy. You have
to be real strong 'cause chemotherapy will knock you down, if
you're standing on all fours, it will still knock you down. I'd
tell him what I go through. I won't try to prepare him for what
he's in for, what I prepare him for what he wants to know, I
tell him what I feel. Certain things, like my bladder, is all
messed up from the chemotherapy, I only urinate once it's full
and then I let it out. I would tell him everything that is going
to happen and to take it one day at a time, and then after I tell
him all this, and whatever he asks me I would try to best tell
him. That when it's all done, hopefully, you'll go home for

good, and when it's all done you just want to put it behind you and go on with the rest of your life.

When you're sick, everything stops. When it's in your leg, it's difficult because that stops you from walking, you can't do everything you want to because once it's in your legs, that's it. You can't do everything that normally you could do, it's like a handicap. You have to go back to another life, like starting all over again. I can't get up and play football like I used to. When you have cancer all of this is just something you have to learn to live with and just take it one day at a time, don't bother to worry about what's gonna happen today or tomorrow, just be happy, think what's coming in your future, like maybe your mother and father are planing a trip. I'm just looking forward, day by day, month by month, and I can look forward to that trip, and not really deal with what's gonna happen because I know what's gonna happen.

That really depresses a lot of people when your hair falls out like, "Oh no, my hair, of all things why my hair." But you know it's gonna happen, and you can hope it's not gonna happen to you because there are one or two patients whose hair does not fall out. Before I got treatment, they told me there was one kid who got chemotherapy and nothing happened to him, he never got sick, his hair never fell out. In the beginning you're like, "I hope I don't get sick. I hope I'm just like that one in a million kid." That's what a lot of patients do because most of the nurses tell you that. You're hoping out of that one hundred or one thousand that that just may be you, but that's not the case when it happens. It's very, very sickening to go through.

This other guy and I, he and I started out at the same time. He had the same thing I had in my leg. I have it from the knee cap up, he has it from the knee cap down. I have it on the right leg, he has it on the left leg. We were going through everything, and believe it or not, we used to live on the same block.

I was in the middle of the block and he was at the corner, and I remember when I was small, I broke his window, and when we met at the hospital, he was like, "Yo, you, you broke my window." That's when everything started happening, that's when my mother met his mother, and everything started to happen. His sickness and my sickness was the same, so when everything started, we came here, we spoke to the doctor and that's when they told us about the different tests we had to go through, having the operation itself, having a bone transplant, going through the physical therapy and all that, bending the leg. It's not so much a problem, bending it.

My biggest dream is to go back and learn to drive a bike again.

They only understand

what I tell them

About a month ago, they told me that I had this malignant tumor in my leg, that I'd get chemotherapy, and a lot of tests. It's been really hard. I was confused, I was, like, "Why does it have to happen to me?" I was like, "What did I do? I'm young." But I just, you know, felt like I was very young, you know, I had a good summer. The next thing I knew I was hit with cancer and, like, it was really shocking to me. It wasn't fun. It was like something hit you all at once. It's like you don't know what to do first. And then, it was just very hard. It's still hard, you know, dealing with the operation, knowing that I'm going to have a metal prosthesis put in my leg, and then I'm going to have a scar, and walking will be hard for me, and losing my hair. I couldn't believe it. It was like, "Oh my God." It's very, very, it's scary.

When I first found out that I had to take chemo for a year, knowing that I had to constantly be in the hospital, knowing that I was gonna constantly get sick and not feel myself and lose weight, and there was gonna be a lot of pain with the operation, and you know, it was a lot of sickness and pain, and I was just, it was nothing I wanted to deal with right now. But, it was either that or not live any more.

I just take one day at a time. It's like, OK, this is what I'm going to do today. And I don't plan for the future. I don't know what's going to happen in the future, with my chemo and all, OK, next week I'm going to have chemotherapy, but I like just take one day at a time. You know, I don't rush things, and that's about it. I mean, it's still hard for me, I get really depressed. I can sit down and cry, it's like, I still can't believe it, I can't believe it. You know, sometimes I like, I don't want to live any more. I'm tired of this. I'm tired of being sick.

I talk to my mother and my friends and, like, they give me some sort of words of confidence, and it's OK, like, "Be glad you're having this or you wouldn't be living right now," you know? It's like, yeah, it's kind of worth it, when you think about it like that. But sometimes, on the other hand, it's like, you don't want to go through with it, it's like, you don't want to come here every week and do this.

What I don't understand is, everybody's like, "I understand what you're going through," but no, nobody understands what I'm going through because they're not going through it, and I don't like that. I like when they say, "OK, I could try to understand what you're going through," but they don't feel the pain that I feel. They only feel the pain that I feel when I'm hurt, and they're hurt. But they don't feel anything else, you know, when I feel physical pain, they feel emotional. It's like, I hate when they say, "Oh, I understand, I understand exactly what you're going through." You've been through it and they haven't, and I don't like that. I don't like that at all. It's like, you understand that it's OK to be bald? It's not, you know? Understand that I had this big operation. It's too hard. They only understand what I tell them.

I had a boyfriend who left me, because he knew that I was going to lose my hair and not look the same for a year. And it hurt so much. It hurts. It's like so painful inside. You don't know what to do with yourself any more. I was only going out with him five months before I found out I had cancer. And it's just like fine, you know, he only went out with me for what I look like. Like, he didn't notice what was on the inside. And then, I just, I don't know, it's just like, hard, that's all I can say. He said, "I don't want to go out with you any more because you're not going to have any hair, and you can't go out on Friday and Saturday nights, and you can't dance. I want to be with someone that could dance, and who has hair, and doesn't look like what you're gonna look like." I said, "Thank you. Thank you, I appreciate that." It hurt a lot. I think it hurt more than anything else. Like, when I needed him the most, why would he want to leave me? But you know, I guess he's kind of young.

Nothing has changed between my friends. I mean, we're still as close as we were. They accept the fact that I have cancer and that I look a little different and I can't really be with them as much. But they've been really supportive about it, I mean, they call me all the time when I'm in the hospital. They try to make it over as much as possible to see me. And they feel terrible for me, and really upset. As long as they're strong, I'm strong too. I'm still their friend, and you know, they just give me a lot more support. They helped me get pretty much half-way through the chemo and the operation, and they would just tell me that everything's going to be OK, "It's OK, you're going to live." It's a real supporting thing. It's great when you talk to them on the phone, just to hear them say everything's going to be OK.

And they're right behind me. When I'm upset, they get upset too. When I'm happy, they're happy. Most of the time they cheer me up. They still tell me their problems all the time, and I help them out, too. They're still the same, it's just like, they're a lot more—I don't know how to say it—they're there a lot more than they would usually be. I mean, my friends were always there with me, hanging out and having a good time, but they're there a lot more for me now.

My family, they've been really great about it, but, it's like, I can't explain it. They've been good, they've been really good. I mean, they're trying to hide their feelings, but I know, my mother's ready to pass out already. She can't do it any more. She's like getting so tired, the running back and forth. I mean, my mom, she's not really that well. And, she's tired. She's exhausted from everything. Constantly staying in the hospital with me, she's missing a lot of work, and that, you know, she needs the money to support me and the house. She's been great, though. I think the parents are more sensitive than the kids. I think they're more hurt than we are. For us, you know, we don't get as emotional. 'Cause I remember my mother cried every night. Well, I was like, there's nothing we can do, you know, I didn't cry every night. And she couldn't concentrate at work. I don't understand why she couldn't concentrate at work. I should be the one who couldn't concentrate, I should be the one who cried all night 'cause I was nervous, but it was her. She was, I think they're more sensitive because we're their children and they can't stand to see us go through it.

They've all been so strong for me. They've been really good. My brother's a little tight, I mean, everything has to be in the mind. Like, he thinks that if you think positive, everything will go away. If you think positive, the pain will go away. If you think positive about—you know, everything has to be, think positive. And it's not always like that. It's like, not to think negative about anything or about yourself or bring yourself down. Like, "You can always do it, you can do it, you can do it." And it's like, I can't always do it. "Yes you can," and then I get into an argument with him. It's like, everything is mind power. Your mind controls everything. I didn't like that at all. I mean, I had a lot of pain during my operation. And he's like, think positively, and the pain will go away. No, the pain did not go away. That was like the most painful thing I ever went through. I can't really think positive, you know.

Because if I do, it still doesn't work for me. Like, give me some aspirins. But he's been good too.

My nephew has been great, out of all of them. He found out that I had to go for chemotherapy and we had to sit him down and explain to him exactly what I'm going through, and that I'm not going to be home all the time, and that I'm going to lose my hair and I don't want him to be shocked when he sees me. My nephew turns around and goes, "Well, I want to go bald too." He did it for me, he shaved his head, down to a crewcut, very short, it was great, you know, it was like, "Wow, I'm gonna be just like you." And he doesn't want his hair to grow back until mine grows back. And he's been great, he does things for me, he's very helpful. He's been really good. He's a good kid. He tries to understand, he's constantly talking about me in school. You know, he comes home, it's like, "Oh this, that, my aunt this, my aunt that." The kids are sick of it already. They're like, "I don't want to hear it any more." But he's a fun kid. We joke around about losing my hair. It's really funny. When I came home from the hospital I said, "OK, I'm going to show you my leg." He took two steps backwards. He was like, "Whoa, what are those things in your leg?" I said, "Staples, they're coming out today." So he said, "Oh, great, good, good." He was really happy for me. So I let him touch my leg and I let him feel the difference between the two legs. He's like, "Wow." He was really amazed by it.

They all deal with it in their little ways. They don't really express any feelings to me of how they feel. My mom will go downstairs and cry. My brother will take it out on being very moody. My sister-in-law? I haven't really seen her emotions. The only time I saw her emotions was when my hair fell out, at the dinner table, clumps of hair, and everybody was in shock, they were sitting around the table. And, uh, she started crying, when I had to lose my hair. Yeah, I was right in the middle of dinner. And so what we did, we were like, "Well, let's get rid of it." And well, "Why are we gonna be depressed for another couple days?" I went downstairs to the basement, and we all took turns cutting away at my hair. And I just wore my wig after that. I was like, "Why am I going to wait for all my hair to fall out, and be depressed about it, let me get it over with now, and cry tonight, and that's it." And I cried 'cause like, when I was young, I always had short hair, and I've always wanted long hair, and it took me like so long to finally get it to where I wanted it. And it was just at that point where I wanted it, you know, I had a nice style and everything. Next thing you know, it's my hair's gone. I'm gonna have to work so hard again to get it to where it was. But, it's been an experience, it's really been an experience. It's so different from what anybody else has been through.

It's changed me a lot. I understand more. I can see things a lot differently. Like, if I never had cancer, and I saw a bald child with cancer, I would kind of be in shock. But it's just these things that like, other sixteen-year-olds wouldn't see, if you know what I mean. Like, I'll analyze a situation more, I wouldn't give you such a quick answer. Like, if you told me to think about something, if I never had cancer, I'd give you a dumb answer within, like, a minute. Now I would sit down and think about it and try to give you a really good answer, and work really hard about it. About anything, it doesn't have to be about cancer. Before, I'd give you a stupid answer, and laugh and walk away. But that was me, you know, it's like everything was fun and games for me. It's like, OK, I plan for the weekend, I plan for a test in school, and that's about it. You know, it's like nothing was ever serious with me. But now it's like, everything's down to earth. I'm more mellowed out. I don't want to go out as much, I don't want to party as much. It's not worth it any more, like, I'm not into that. I'm now more into getting ahead at school, and I'm looking towards the future for my life. You know, well I have my life now, if I get to go on, well, I'm gonna make something out of it. Just to go on, and to make something out of myself. I'm planning to go to college, and just to keep going, and work really hard.

I can't wait, I'm just waiting for this to end. I'd rather be in school. I mean, I'm home all the time, laying in bed, watching the TV. There's nothing for me to do any more. And my friends are in school. I think that's what depresses me the most. Like, I can't be with the people I want to be with when I want to. And like, nobody's home with me, and nobody to talk to. I just twiddle my thumbs all day, and I think that's what depresses me the most, besides being here. I mean, the operation's over, it's great, now I'm just working to walk again, working really hard. And the chemo, it's like I'm used to the chemo already, so I really have no problem with that. It's just like I don't want to do it any more, but I have no other choice.

Like I talk to some of the other kids in the hospital and it really scares me. I mean, I'm happy for them. I like to know what they went through, what I'm gonna go through. It's like, I would get different answers from a doctor, the doctor would give me, like, not full answers, you know, and the kids would give me exactly what they felt, what they went through, and it's a lot better.

I met one kid who had, um, a metal plate put in his arm, cause he had a tumor, and uh, a couple months later he found out that he had cancer in his joints, and his arm, and they amputated his arm, and now he's back with something else in his stomach. So that kind of scared me, thinking about, "Wow, am I going to have cancer again, is it going to come back?" It's a scary thought, knowing I have cancer and that it'll probably come back. And I don't want to think about it. I just wanna go on, just forget about it. It's kind of scary to think it's going to come back, you know. I hope the chemo works, and cures everything.

I have this other friend that I met here and, um, he has, uh, cancer of the bone marrow, in his hip, and he's going to go through a really fatal operation where they're going to take out the bone marrow in that part of his body, and, um, and like, he may not survive this operation, because he's getting really strong chemo put into his body, and they took out, I can't really remember what he said to me, but I know they were taking something out of his body, that he wouldn't be with for about a week or so, and then they have to inject it back in. It's a really strong chemo, and he's going to be in isolation and everything. He's worse off than I am. He told me that he may not survive, that's what he told me. He was really open with me. This is the first time I met him. We were very open with each other, about how we felt. I went to him crying one day and he told me, "Don't cry, you know, it's OK." He's been through a lot more than I've been through, and he's been in the hospital for three months and he's such a nice kid. I pray for him all the time.

Last Friday, I was in the hospital for my operation, and I was getting ready to leave Saturday, but I was so anxious to get out of the hospital that I had to leave that day. I didn't care if nobody came to pick me up, I was going to hop into a cab and leave here, bring all my stuff back. I got dressed, thinking that I'm going to leave, you know, and I went there, screaming and crying at the top of my lungs, "I've gotta get out of here, my life is ruined, everything is ruined!" And my doctor, she started crying, because I got so upset. I was just throwing all my depression out on her. Tears, her eyes started watering up, and she's like, "I know, I know, I know, it's hard." I was like, "No. No. You don't know anything. You just don't know anything." I was like, "Look at my leg, look at me, I'm bald and disgusting-looking." 'Cause I was always worried about my appearance when I had hair and every-thing, everything had to be perfect on me. Yeah, that's the way it is, you know, you're a teenager and especially if you're a girl. And now it's like, God, nobody's going to look at me. You know, I was like going crazy.

And then, I started laughing after a while. I was like, forget it, I'm giving myself a major headache, my blood pressure must be like, so high. I was ready to pass out already. I was just like, forget it. Why am I going to get so upset? I'm not going to do that any more. Whenever I freak out, they want to put me on Valium, sleeping pills, and I was like, no way, I can deal with this myself, I don't need drugs to make me calm. I mean, just let it happen naturally. Then I'm just gonna rely on drugs to keep me calm and I don't want that. You know, I don't like drugs at all.

I scare very easily, and the staff tells me things like, they tell me something, but they don't tell me like, the gory details, so they're honest with me up until a certain point, and then it stops. Sometimes I get that feeling, like, something's not right, you know, when they sit down and tell me, you know, what pain, or, anything about pain or, it's going to work well, or you know it's like, well, I don't like it. Like, I feel like something's wrong, they're not going to tell me everything. But then sometimes I don't want to hear everything they have to say because then I get paranoid, like, oh my God, and I can't go through that.

Like, um, I was getting my broviac[1] put in, one week, and, I was getting my first dose of, um, adriamycin, and like, that's the strongest medicine I ever got. And I was pushed into having a broviac and three days of chemo in one week. I went home sick for almost two weeks. And I didn't think that I should be pushed into something, like I never have a say any more of what I want to do. I mean I have a story about how I feel, but it's not, I don't have the way to like, say stop, or, I want a break from this already. It's like I'm always being pushed into something that I don't feel like doing at that point. I mean, they hear me out, but they don't care. It's like you have to get this broviac and you have to have chemo. I was sick. I couldn't hear, my neck was tilted to the side, I hunched over, I had headaches, I couldn't get out of bed for at least three days 'til my mother dragged me out of bed. I lost my appetite, I slept all day, and it was terrible, and I was so mad at them for doing that to me. I mean, why couldn't they give me the broviac one week, and let me rest the following week. I didn't think that was fair.

Everybody has a right to know what's going on in their life. I mean, I would be kind of upset if someone just gave me medicine and I don't know why they're giving me medicine, why they're doing this. I want to know before you inject something into me. If I don't know what you're giving me, I have to know. I'm like that. I have to watch everything that they do. I have to know everything, 'cause I don't trust people sometimes. That's what I tell the other kids here. I tell them things that people have told me, that it's really hard, and you just gotta deal with it, you know, you really have no other choice, unless you don't want to live any more, and I'm sure you want to live. So I guess you have to sacrifice a year out of your life or not have a life at all. And it's kind of rotten if you think about it. It's one year, rather than nothing at all, and I'm willing to sacrifice that one year out of my life. I'm willing to sacrifice every piece I have of my body just to live. At first I wasn't willing to do that, and now it's like, I'd give up anything just to live, and I don't care. You know, as long as I have my life, it's fine with me.

One month later

I was supposed to come in for chemo last Wednesday but on Tuesday night I decided not to go in. I didn't want to go in at all 'cause I was fed up with it. I was tired, I'm sick of this. I hate it and I don't want to do it any more. And I didn't go in and my mother called up and said that I wasn't showing up, and they threatened to get a court order against me, saying that I was under age. I'm tired of people making decisions for me. They speak for me, they answer for me, I never could say anything, 'cause I'm underage. I'm still a human, I'm allowed to make decisions.

Sometimes I want to die, believe me. I didn't care about anything, I mean, I don't care about anything, at all. 'Cause if I did care, I would come in for chemo, I would let them do my leg. But I don't care any more. I just don't care about anything that happens. I'm only sixteen. I don't want to do this anymore. I took a year out of my life. Everyone says, "Well, there's a lot more years ahead of you, so you're gonna be missing one year, big deal." But it's not like that any more. I can't do anything. I'm constantly in this place, and I don't want to be here anymore. I'm tired of getting sick. I was thinking like they could put you to sleep, right, and wake you up when it's all over with, getting the treatments and everything. And they can't do that, freeze you or something. I know I have to have it. It's like, I wanna do it, like I want to get the treatment, 'cause I know I do want to live. On the other hand it's like, "No, I don't want this treatment at all, I don't care if I live, I don't care if I die."

I hate getting sick. I don't like the way I look any more. That bothers me, too. You know, I look at my girl friends, their hair, and they dye it, and I want to dye my hair, and I wanna spray it up, and I can't do that any more, and I'm getting pissed. I can't do anything. I've got to be here in this hospital, I want to go to school, I can't do that, I want to be with my friends, I can't. I mean, I can do that, but not as often as I would. I just want to be myself again.

I don't want to talk to these doctors anymore. I give them snappy answers. I don't like them. I don't know why, they're nice people, I just, I don't like them. And they're telling me that they're—I had a doctor come in yesterday, and he told me that he was busting his ass for me. What is he doing? He doesn't have any physical contact with me, he's not doing anything to me. All he's doing, he's not even putting the medicine in me, you know, connecting it to me. So how is he busting his ass? I don't understand that, there's no physical contact. I mean, I could see if you're doing something to me, physically, but you're not. The chemo is doing it all by itself. So I don't know where they came up with that. All they probably do is sit back in their offices.

Did you talk to anybody who was like me, going through what I'm going through, I mean, like, feeling what I'm feeling? Have you talked to a lot of girls? I don't know, sometimes I think the girls like, um, how do I explain it? I can't get that word out, um, oh God, I can't get it out. That girls take it much harder than the guys. The guys take it like, "Oh, it's OK," you know, they can still go out and play football, whatever. And we're like, we take it like it's something like, "Oh my God." We get depressed about it. I don't think the guys get like that. They take it very lightly, the way they show it. They take it like it's nothing. They, like, don't express their feelings to me, like, "Yeah, you know, big thing, so I'm here, I'm here, big deal." For me it's like, "Big Deal." I don't want to be here. I don't understand that. I speak to the guys here but they never mention about how they feel, I mean, I sit there and spill my heart out. Three days, chemo, big deal. Ugh, I hate it. I can't relate to them, you know. I mean, how come you feel like that and I feel like this?

Like this one guy, he had a relapse. He's taking it well. I would have been like, "No, no more." I think he's putting up a really good front, and I think at nighttime, he must have his moments, I know I would. I bet you he's hurting. He just doesn't want to show it. I'm sure he sits in his room and gives a little cry here and there, 'cause I know I would, I would lose it totally, to have to come back here. The fact of coming back, going through it again would drive me bananas. I'm just scared that it's gonna come back. People are different in the way that they show their feelings. I handle my feelings in one way and I feel that's good for me, and he may feel that's good for him. He takes it so easy, that's the way it seems to me. It's not easy, but they put up such a front, like it's no big thing, but me, I've got to express my feelings straight out.

These guys, I know some of them do worry about the way they look and their hair, but I think it's harder on a girl to deal with not having hair, they can't deal with it. I guess a girl has to look a certain way. We get really insecure about ourselves when we don't look right. Lately, I've been pretty insecure. Like, "OK, I look fine, I look good. No, I look disgusting." It's a really weird experience, "Wow, no hair." It's really weird. It's different, just looking like this. I bought a wig for five hundred dollars and wore it for maybe two weeks, and I threw it in the bag. It wasn't me. I knew from the start that a wig is just not me, it's not my hair. I walked around thinking everyone was looking at me and knows it's not real. You could tell, it's got like that plastic look to it, it's ugly. It just wasn't me, it wasn't what I wanted, it wasn't the right color.

Wherever I walked everyone looked at me, it's hard to know what they're looking at, everyone looks at me, looks at my leg. It bothers me because I'm so curious, "Why are you looking at me?" I want to know what they're thinking. I think they would probably say they wondered what happened to me, try to figure out these bad things I have.

What I'm feeling, is it normal? I don't know. Is it OK to feel like this? I mean, does everybody else feel like this? You know what I mean? It's like, is it OK to feel like this? Should I feel any other difference? I guess it's normal. I guess the way you feel about anything is normal. It's natural, right? I mean, is it OK to feel like this? Like the anger and depression. Like they tell me that there's no need to feel depressed, you know. That's a bunch of BS, OK? No need to feel depressed? Why don't you go for some chemotherapy and have your bone removed and have complications with it. No, there's no need to be depressed. That doesn't make sense. I mean, if I wasn't depressed I don't think I'd be normal. Nobody can explain to me why I shouldn't be depressed, they just don't want to see me depressed.

My brother says, "You're depressed and you don't know about it," my mother says that I shouldn't be depressed, and my sister-in-law doesn't say a word. I think they're just as confused as I am. Like, I'm happy one minute, mad the next. The nurses think I'm schizo. It's really unusual for me to be happy, when I'm here, I know that. And I came on Monday very happy for some reason. The nurses thought it was really strange. I walked around dancing and singing a song. But that doesn't last, my moods change very quickly. It just happens, you don't even know when it happens.

I had a dream that the doctor called up and said it was really unusual if I lost my hair, and I already lost my hair. A couple of days after the operation I had a dream that I was skating very fast, and I crashed into a wall, and I stuck my bad leg out on purpose to like smash it up. I was pretty angry I guess. I think I was probably mad at my leg or something. It was like I don't care, I was banging it into the wall. I had a dream that I was locked in a refrigerator and there was a window where I could see out but they couldn't see in, and I could hear them, but they couldn't hear me, and I was slowly dying because of the oxygen. I was using up too much oxygen. That was weird. I was real scared when I woke up. That's the strangest dream I had, being locked in a refrigerator. Then there was one dream

I had that I was stuck on top of a ferris wheel, up there in the middle of nowhere, and it was dark, and it was cold, and I just sat up there. I had a dream last night that I was a taxi cab driver, and I drove for six hours straight. I remember picking up passengers, I just don't know who they are, and I forgot to punch out to get paid, and I missed two days of pay.

It's nothing. It's no big deal

I found out I have cancer in my knee about three weeks ago. A doctor at my school told me and it was no surprise. I'm aware of cancer and stuff. I talked to my friend, I talked to everybody about it. He told me how I have a possibility of getting a tumor, a cancer tumor. This to me is no, it's not a big deal because it's treatable, you know, it's an illness. They quote this survey, I don't know if it's sure, that one out of four Americans get cancer. I read that in a book, I'm not sure if it's true, but I mean that's kinda high, so to me it's no big deal, and the treatment's only ten months. I feel kind of sad in a way, like I wouldn't say unfortunate but, you know, I don't question myself and say, "Why is it me?" "Why not me?" It could happen to anybody. And the only thing I feel sad about is that I'll miss school. That's about it.

And my parents get a little worried and everything but the doctors explained everything. Like the ten months of treatment, um, like the first two months, it's like chemotherapy, and then I'll have surgery. They said that in the surgery they'll cut out, like a piece of my tibia below my kneecap and replace it with, um, titanium, I believe it was. They said that during the surgery they will find out if I need a new knee, because they don't know how long my knee's been exposed to cancer, whatever. And after surgery, I have another eight months of chemotherapy. And what they said is, I, most people'll be back in their normal life. And I don't know if it's true or not, like, it's not genetically caused. So to me it's nothing. I hopefully can go on with my life after the treatment and go back and continue on with my life. It's no big deal, I mean, to me. It's a setback, that's about it.

The one big thing is that I'm an athlete. I play like virtually every sport in the book. And what I'm going to lose later on, after the surgery and this stuff, is that I cannot run. I mean they say I cannot even play tennis and I cannot ski for my life. That is a big thing. I cried when I heard that, but then they say I could play other sports instead of that sport, but that's a big thing, that's what I'll miss a lot. But what can I do? You know it wouldn't kill me not to play tennis, 'cause I've been playing it for like the last eight years. And I'm a big fan, but if I can't play it, I'll watch it then. It's no big deal to me. I'll find a new sport, swimming or golf, whatever.

They broke the news to me first, and then they broke the news to my mom. My mom and my aunt were there and they cried and stuff. I told them in advance, already, I might have cancer, so my relatives were behind me, in front and behind me. I told everyone I knew that I have cancer. I mean it's only an illness. And my friends, I'd see them in school, like two days ago I saw them in school, and they're very supportive, that's what's great about it. They say they feel sorry for me. They say, "You'll be back in school and stuff in no time." It's only a year, you know. I don't want them to say, "Oh Jesus, why is it you?" I don't want them to pray and I don't want them to be too sorry for me, or anything like that.

This girl, like we've been going out, not actually a girlfriend, like we've been going out and stuff. I told her I had cancer and she kind of cried, and she's kind of mad at me because, um, because, not because I have cancer, but because I joke around a lot, that I took this as a joke. Well, this is not a joke, it's deadly, but she's mad because I joke around. She cried. She didn't tell me that she was mad at me, she just told my best friend and stuff. What can I do? I mean, I got cancer, I come here for treatment, I'm not going to feel depressed about it. Maybe I cried a couple times. I don't reflect on it, I don't look back and say, "Why me?" I don't do that. But I cried like twice, I think, I mean like, you know, to myself. I don't want to cry in front of my mom. I want to be strong I guess. I'm not a strong or tough guy or anything, but I don't want my mother—like, I feel that if I cry, if I look so sad you know, like, don't do this, don't do that, what I used to do normally, that'd make my mom even worse. So I don't do that.

Before I had cancer I didn't know very much about it. People should be more aware of cancer. When I got cancer, I found out so much about medicine. I mean the facts, this, that, you know. Even if you don't have cancer, you can be aware of it. The problem with people who have cancer is, like people ask you, and you have to explain to them what is this, what is that, you know. Not many people would seem to know, you know. I explain to them, I'm open, I could talk about cancer, it doesn't hurt me to talk about it.

The nurses and the doctors, they're very nice and like, I mean, I don't know. I don't go to the hospital that much but these people seem very nice. I think that the best way to treat a patient is to have a good sense of humor and joke around a little.

I miss school, that's the biggest thing I'm missing. Because most of the time, like, I spent time studying a lot so, but here I've been doing nothing but sitting around, and reading books. It's not like studying any more, so I don't know. Sometimes I think it's a waste of time, just sitting here, but it's not, it's the treatment. They tried to put me in the bone scan, like for fifteen minutes, because of my leg, I couldn't stretch it out before. It was kind of painful but I can take it. They tried to put me under the MRI scan, which is the magnetic resolution images. They tried putting me in for an hour, but I said forget it, my leg won't take it. I know I'd be in pain. It's painful when I stretch my legs out for five or ten minutes, so I'd skip it.

Seriously, I'm not afraid of cancer because someone could be worse, I mean like, people drive a car, I mean like, you figure, your chances of getting killed isn't so high. Sometimes I do bad in school, like, not that bad, bad on one test I studied and I did bad on it. I feel really mad and I want to kill myself. Why me? Why did I do so bad in school, you know. I'm sure everyone, I don't know about everybody but I had a feeling that—you know, of suicide, like you know, before, I guess because of school, because school is the biggest thing for me. School is the thing, I have to be successful in school because everybody in my family is college-oriented. And you know, I thought, before, I thought of death before anything was going. Even if I studied for an exam and I did bad on it, maybe I got a D or E you know, something like that. I compare that to cancer.

The biggest thing, if I were to die because of cancer, I mean that's possible you know, um, but I think the biggest thing, the people, you know, like my family, are the ones being pained more than I am, who get hurt the most. They're suffering more than I do. The doctor told my parents that it's not your fault, it's not anyone's fault, it's cancer, and it's not genetic. Maybe, I don't know. Because my mom, she's coming over here almost every day. She worries about me very much.

After this week my hair should be falling out. Um, it's no big thing to me. I mean it's no big thing, it's only ten months, make it a year. I mean other people who are going bald, those are permanent. What I have is just temporary. Some people, I see some people who get their hair shaved off, it's no big thing to me, you know. I've never had my hair shaved or anything like that but it's no big deal, it's only ten months. I could handle that, I mean, just wear a hat, a baseball cap. That's a big thing for a lot of people. Like, um, to me it's not a big thing because I told my friends, like I'm going to have chemotherapy and my hair will be falling out, and they said, "But what will happen to your hair? I mean, will your hair fall out that much?" And I told them everything. So that's a side effect. I won't have hair, and I told them, so later on they won't be surprised. So it's no big thing any more, it's no big deal. Maybe having your hair fall out will make you less socialized in a group of crowded people or something like that. Maybe it'll stop you from going to a party, or going out to the movies, but I don't think that it'll keep me from doing it. I'll just keep doing what I do all my life.

Two months later, on the day before surgery

They told me it was only going to be one surgery, just for the knee. And it's fine, you know, I was looking forward to it. Then yesterday, the doctor told my parents and myself about the possibility of lung surgery. So now I have two surgeries to look forward to instead of one, and one is okay, but two, to me I never had surgery before and it's a big thing, you know. It's kind of upset me so much, I mean, I cried so much and if, only if they could tell me later, I mean after the first surgery, to tell me about the lung surgery so I wouldn't have suffered so much. You know, OK, what the hell, it's only another surgery, let's get it over with. Now, you know, it's too much.

But the reason she told me now instead of telling me after the first one was because I'll be more awake and conscious to know what it is. I'd be more able to understand, if I have any question for them. But I was really mad yesterday. Today I'm, you know, it's the day after, and I'm kind of seeing that it's okay, that I have no choice but to get on, just get the surgery over with. My mom and dad told me, "Don't worry," you know, God be with me, "Just pray that it's not a tumor. Whatever it is, they have to take it out anyway, so don't worry. Just look on the positive side, try to look on the bright side."

I try to think that it's only another surgery, they just put me to sleep and then take it out. The only thing about surgery is before the surgery, you go through all these tests and everything. It's the waiting and everything. It's really, like this thing, it's all in the mind. It's really made me think, you know. As the day gets closer to surgery, it's harder for me to go to sleep, you know. Before it was like fine, and the last couple days, it's hard for me to go to sleep. It's taken me an hour or two longer to go to sleep. At nighttime I think about it, think about what they're going to do to me and how I'm going to feel after surgery, and how I'm going to deal with the prosthesis that will be in my leg, and losing all my ability to walk, you know, and stuff.

I really don't care about the lung surgery. It's just another cut in my body, and they're going to take it out. Either I have it or I don't have it. They're going to cut it up and take a look anyway, so what's the big deal, you know, if they're going to cut it up and I have it, they're going to take it out, or I don't have it, they're going to take out the dead cells anyway, so it doesn't make any difference anyway. But the leg surgery, I mean, they made me sign a consent yesterday, saying that I gave the hospital consent to remove my knee and replace it with a prosthesis, and at the end, it said, as the last resort, it's to be amputated, you know. Then I would think twice. I asked the doctor, what does it mean, you know? That's scary, there. I hope everything goes well. The odds are in my favor, but it's that last thing, it made me think twice, three times about, you know, amputation. I mean that's the last thing I want to do, you know, and I don't know how I'd deal with that, amputating. I'd rather not go on living. I don't think I could survive with my leg being cut off, I mean for me, it's a big thing. That would be too much for me to handle. Even to talk about amputation would make me cry, you know, it's hard for me. But I hope that everything goes well tomorrow. I adjusted to the fact that I'm going to get a prosthesis in my knee, you know. At least I'll be able to walk.

As time moves on, I deal with the cancer much better. I told myself it's just, you know, before I came to the hospital, before I came in yesterday, I was saying it's only another surgery. After surgery I'll feel much better. And then they say it's only eight more months of chemotherapy and I have two months already. And it's not a big thing, you know. I mean I survived the two months so I tell myself I can survive another eight months of chemo. Even though I have a little trouble with it, you know it's the toughest thing in my life. The chemical that's going into my body makes me feel really sick and makes me vomit all the time, and I can't eat and stuff, you know. If I ever can't eat I get really tired, and if I can't eat for three or four days, then when I get home I'm like helpless, you know. I can't move around, and I hate that, you know, because I'm an active person and I hate to, not to move around. I mean I'm really scared of being weak. But I'm adjusting to it, to the level of it.

OK, I say, it's only three or four days of it and I'll be fine, you know, as the day goes on. I have three days of chemotherapy and then the fourth day at home. I get helpless, I mean, in my whole life, I mean I never depended on anybody. I've never been in the hospital in my life before I got cancer. And it's scary because I mean I, I don't know what to say, I mean like, it's so sudden. You know like, I don't know, I mean it was scary, I mean I'm afraid I won't last, you know. Like before, I mean at home, three days of chemotherapy, the fourth or fifth days I cannot move, I cannot eat, and I feel like I'm dying. I mean I say, is it really worth living, you know? I mean this thing has really gotten to me. I mean I've thought about dying and stuff, you know. That's up to that point, you know. I really don't know what to say, but I mean, the suffering is so tremendous that I, it is, maybe it's easier for me to die then to live on and to deal with the pain and the agony of it, you know. Maybe it's just easier to die than to live on.

I may not make it. I think if I die, it's just easier for me, you know, just a long sleep, that's all. It's no big thing to me, you know. I think I'm so young, but I think it's easier. But on the other hand my parents are supportive and stuff. They just told me to keep up the spirit. All the other patients I've looked at, they've always survived, they just suffer for a short time, but they survive. Before, when I talked to you, the last time I was, I believe I told you it's no big thing about cancer, I believe I said that. Now I changed my mind, that it is a big thing. It is the worst. Before when I met you, I told you it's no big thing, it's just a setback, that's the word I used. Now it's suffering and I know I can really die from this, you know, I don't know, I mean, I think to kill myself and stuff. I really can't die because it's hard for my parents and family to accept. I don't want to make them feel bad. I don't know because, I mean, dying, for me is OK, but I think it's a big thing for my parents because I saw how my mom felt when my grandpa just passed away like a month ago. Because it's so hard for her. I know how hard it is for her to have a son pass away.

The nurses are great here, even the doctors. I think everybody in this hospital are very nice, you know. They talk and they're very nice, I mean, I can't ask for anything else from other people. They're the greatest people around. I mean, I can't ask for more. Everybody tries to make me, I mean all I could ask from them is being nice, and they are being so nice to me. I can't ask for more, especially the doctor that takes care of me, the nurses, everybody's been nice.

I know I'll have problems falling asleep tonight, there's no doubt about it. But then they'll give me, I'll ask for like a drug, it made me fall asleep last night. So I'll just go to sleep and wake up in the morning, and go down to the surgery room, and I hope they don't make me wait, because I think waiting's the worst thing in the hospital. It makes me think, you know, and I don't want to think about it. Hopefully there's not much pain afterwards, but they'll give me a painkiller, so I can fall asleep.

I really don't know how I feel, you know, when the day comes for the lung surgery, I really don't know how I'm going to deal with that. But I'll take one at a time. I don't have a choice now. This thing is just like, well, they give me choice A, now let's do it and I must take choice A, no other choice not to accept it. I try to deal with it because you feel you have no choice but to accept what they tell you. I'm sure they do the best they can, and so I take their word for it. But I guess it's difficult for me to accept the lung surgery. I guess before this, they could not find this spot on the CAT scan, and it's making me wonder, how come it showed up now. And it makes me even further wonder if they see that spot now, what happens if they take my CAT scan like two months from now, and I'm wondering what'll happen if they see some more, you know, like dots, some more bone tumor in other parts of my body. It's hard for me to accept that.

I mean, first my knee, you know, I accepted that, and I said OK, it's just the knee. Now the lung. Now I try to adjust, OK, it's just the knee and the lung. And hopefully it won't be any more. Hopefully they won't tell me that they found some other spot in another part of my body. That's a big thing I'm hoping for. I hope it's just, the lung is just the end of it. I mean if it shows up in another place, I really don't know what to do. I mean, I'll say forget it. I mean, I took their word for it, you know. I took their word for it when they said it's just the knee, you know. And now it's just, they kind of lied to me. And I know I cannot blame them for it. I mean, I really cannot, but how can I trust them when they tell me in the first place, it just occurred in the knee, and now it's turned around, turned out to be in my lung also. I mean, how could I trust them, if they just told me it's the knee and the lung now.

I mean, they make me worry. I mean, every day it's, they make me think that, day after day, I mean, it may show up in another part of my body. They see it in the CAT scan but it didn't show up then, they didn't tell me that when they told me about the knee. But they should have, I'm sure it's not their fault. I mean they, it didn't show up then, it didn't show up then. Maybe it was too small then and now it's just a little bit bigger. But how is that possible? If they've been giving me chemotherapy it's supposed to reduce it. On the other hand, they don't know for a fact that it is a tumor yet. It might be a dead cancer, a dead tumor cell. So even if it's a tumor, they're going to take it out, so I really don't have another choice. They're going to have to open up my chest and take a look at it, either way. If it's a dead cell or a live cell, they're going to take it out.

I think, I mean, if I survive cancer, I can do anything in life. It is the hardest thing, and I'm sure any obstacle in my life won't be as big as cancer, not as big as dealing with cancer. I'm sure that any problem in my life I could deal with after this. I think this is the biggest thing in my life and if I could deal with it, if I could survive through this, then I think I'd be more, you know, it'll make me a stronger person. It'll make me think that I can do anything with my life, if I'm a success in dealing with the treatment and everything. And I think I can be a successful person in life. That's how I look at it. I'm sure that this is the worst in life.

I mean, anything I can deal with, but cancer is something I'm helpless. Like, maybe I'll have financial problems in life. That's something I could help myself in, make it better. With cancer, I can't help myself. Right now I'm kind of suffering, I've lost all the fun. I mean, I could remember last year, at this time I'd go fishing, I'd go to the beach every day, I mean, I'd enjoy tennis and the outdoors with my friend. And now I look back and I say I'm losing all this. I'm losing it permanent, you know. I'm sure I won't be playing tennis, or skiing, or something like that.

I think, tennis, I've been playing tennis for over eight years now. I was going to try out for college tennis next year. I'll lose that now. They told me I won't be able to play tennis, and I'll never be able to run, that's a big thing. I used to be a runner, you know. And skiing, that's a big thing, I ski in the winter, and I just picked up the sport and I love it. I love it, even more, even much better than tennis. And it's all gone, down the drain now. But on the other hand, I'm, even if I can't ski, or play tennis, I could go scuba diving I think. That's a good thing they told me. I can go swimming. It'll make me strong, a new sport.

If I cannot run, I cannot be an active person. It'll make me study more, you know, at school, something like that. You have to look at the positive side, the bright side. I really look forward to going back, you know, to go fishing, to go back to the beach, next year. That's what I'm looking forward to. I want to live long to do all this stuff, to continue on, to go back to school, is another thing for me. I'd like to go back to school.

Yea, but before surgery, I'm constantly thinking about surgery. Even if I watch the best movie, or watch the best show on TV, it pops up right there. It pops up right on the screen and I don't even notice it's popping up. Like, I'm watching a TV show and I'm watching it, and it's right there, and I really don't know what I'm watching. I've lost my concentration on the show. It changes to a different subject. It changes back to my thinking about it, about cancer. It doesn't matter how much I try, I can't put it aside. I watch TV, just turn it on, just flipping channels, and I start to notice, so many people talking about cancer. Like the other day, just flipping channels, I saw an interview with people who had cancer. And this stuff, before I had cancer, I never noticed this stuff, you know. The other day, too, I saw—before cancer I wouldn't have noticed this stuff, but now I flip and I saw, you know, the surgery, and it made me stop and watch it and it made me think about cancer.

It's so hard, you know. It's for real. I think the biggest thing right now that I'm worried about is, the biggest thing is, if after the lung surgery, if it's ever going to appear in another place. That's the biggest concern that I can imagine. I mean I just cannot imagine how I'm going to feel. How I'm going to act, you know, if I find out I have cancer in another place. I mean, I really don't know. If it doesn't go well, I'd say forget it, if it makes me go to sleep forever, that's how it goes. But I try to look on the positive side, it's the best doctor so hopefully that'll be the end of it. But if it doesn't go well, I don't know what to say, I really don't know what to do about it, if it'll be worth living if it didn't go well.

I'm always acting upset. I mean I've cried, but I don't know what's after that. That's the biggest thing, you know. I mean I cannot afford to have three or four surgeries. I don't think I can suffer that much. Yesterday I cried in front of my parents, in front of my doctor. I think it's healthy to cry. There's nothing wrong with crying. It gets some of the anxiety out. Lets it out more. I don't cry much, I mean. Before, it didn't matter how much you upset me, but I didn't cry before. But this thing, I told myself, this thing has really upset me, that's why I cry so much.

I just want people to be straight
with me

In the beginning it was hard, but now everything's fine. I'm just getting adjusted to it all and accepting what I have. You know, it wasn't easy accepting it. I mean I didn't know at first what it was, the only thing I was, like, the doctor told me I had, um, leukemia and the first thing I thought of was what my hair was gonna look like, you know. And that was one of the most worries of them all. I didn't even realize, I didn't know what it was or anything. I knew my hair was gonna come out and then it all came out, all of it. It just all started falling out and then when I got the radiation all of it came out. At first it was coming out just from the medicines, but not as much, and then, after the radiation, it came out in clumps. It was very scary.

What was so scary is that I would see things on TV when I was well, before I got sick, I'd see these kids on TV with no hair or anything, like, you know, in the cancer places, in the hospitals and stuff. Kids with cancer and I never realized it could actually happen to me. That I could get cancer and actually look like one of those kids on TV. That you don't think it could happen to you, but it can, and it did. All the time I wondered, "Why me?" I mean, it got to one point, I just like, I'm Catholic and I totally just didn't want anything to do with the religion or God or anything, because one of the things was that I couldn't believe it happened to me, and why? There was no reason. I mean it doesn't come from heritage or anything, it just happens. Why was I picked? You know I went into the hospital and saw all the other kids and I couldn't believe that there could be a God if there were so many young kids that couldn't have done anything, infants, that are so sick.

Well, it got tough, like certain medications that you don't know if you're gonna get sick or not. And then like some of the things they say, like you get sick three hours afterwards and if not, you know, that's what it usually is; but like a couple times, I've been the exceptional case, which was scary. Like, once I took this one medication called Cytoxan and they said don't eat through it or you'll get sick afterwards, like three hours afterwards. And I did eat during it because I was too hungry, 'cause I couldn't eat the night before. And I didn't get sick but then like thirteen hours after and that night I went and ate a full-course meal, and I got sick, vomited something like thirteen times in one night. It's not supposed to take that long to get sick, if you're gonna get sick, and when you're getting sick, it's the worst thing. 'Cause like, you know, you sound like, like almost something that would be like a demon almost. It takes a lot out of you.

The drugs are much worse than the cancer itself. They say that, and it's the truth. It's something that goes with the cancer. But it's the drugs that will cure you so if you didn't take the drugs then the cancer would be much worse than the drugs. The Cytoxan I think was the worst medicine of them all, because I just got so sick and it got to the point where they had to knock me out with, um, with different drugs. I forget the name of the drugs they used.

My mom and dad are always worried, and like now it's pretty bad because like every single thing I want to do, you know, they're more up on everything, you know, with what's going on with me. They're always there. They're always afraid to let me do things, and like, with the medications there's always so much, it's like my mom's on this schedule and she cannot get off of the schedule. She writes down everything. So she has pads of paper from when I first got sick to now. Tonight when we go home she'll mark off all my medications. I mean she's kept up on it like I couldn't believe. And my dad, he's always been there to help through everything, with the spinal taps and everything.

They're great, but I mean, it was more of a shock to them I think than it was to me. I mean they were more, I think, shocked than I was, and they—like now, like say after I'm watching something on television, and something about cancer will come on the TV about kids with leukemia, like, I'll wanna watch it and they'll get mad at me for wanting to watch it. But yeah, I still like to see what's happening to other people. It doesn't bother me at all. They were just both so upset.

I was upset, I was so upset, too, I mean, it was a very scary thing. I mean the things that the medication does to you is horrible. You have mood swings. The things that my parents had to put up with that I did, I mean the mood swings. One minute I'll be happy, one minute I'll be sad, one minute I'll be mad. I mean they said that I would stare out the window for hours, and just stare. I can remember sitting and just staring into space, but it's just like things are going through your head, like what's going on, am I gonna make it to finish the remission? Now I still wonder about it, if I'm gonna be able to make it through. But things have just been going so good that I wouldn't think that it would come back again. But every time I come in, every three months for the spinal tap and the bone marrow, you know, you get on edge. Like if the doctor's gonna come up and tell me it's come back again. And if he says, "Yeah, it's fine," I mean the sighs of relief that come out of my mom and my dad and me, and my brother, when he's here. We're all very nervous now, just coming in just for these things. I get all nervous and tired and everything.

I mean, now, if I get a bloody nose or something, just like that they call the doctor quick, you know. And if I get tired and I'm sleeping a lot, my mom and dad still get concerned. I mean my dad's like, "Why are you always so tired?" Because that was one of my symptoms of having it, I was so tired when I would come home that I would sleep all day and all night, and it was just that that was one of the symptoms, that and bloody noses. And now when I get a bloody nose, it's, I get scared even. Anything happens and I get scared.

The doctors would tell me stuff. I think they told me basically pretty much everything, but sometimes my parents would get mad because I would pry to find out things. But I always found out, one way or another. They didn't want to tell me, and that's one thing that I hate. I wanna know what's going on. I don't care how bad it is, I wanna know what's going on. Like they didn't use the word cancer. I went in and, um, I mean, right away, I knew something was wrong when I was at the hematologist because my mom came out, her nose was bright red from crying. And, um, I mean that right there, she just lost me. And then I walked in, I see my dad in there and he was all upset. He was just pale and just sitting there. I can remember it still. I can remember walking into that office and the feeling I had going into that office. I knew something was definitely wrong, terribly wrong. My mom doesn't just come out like that for no reason. So I went in and, um, the doctor said, you know, you have, um, leukemia. And she said to me, you know, they took a bone marrow from me, and um, you know, that's when they decided it was leukemia.

I didn't know what leukemia was. They didn't say cancer, they said leukemia. The word leukemia is so scary that, in itself, you just, you don't know what's going on. You go into a state of shock. I think I went into a state of shock when I heard what I had. It seemed like it was not happening to me. You know what I'm saying? It was like a nightmare. I couldn't talk about it, but now I could talk about it for hours. But before then I didn't know anything. I didn't know, when you see the kids on TV, you don't know, nobody knows anything about what leukemia is, what they're going through unless they go through it. And no one's family will know unless the whole family goes through it.

My parents didn't let me read anything about it because they said, "No, no, no, you don't want to read this, you don't want to read this. This was written a long time ago and it doesn't have updated information and it's all wrong. Don't worry, you don't want to read it." I did want to read it. I did want to know what was going on. They didn't want me to, so I didn't and I don't think I read anything on it. They were hiding stuff from me, and I hate when they hide stuff from me. I hate that more than anything. I just want people to be straight with me on what's going on. So I talked to the doctor and I would ask him stuff when they weren't around. Who would tell me? I think, I don't know, maybe they told him not to tell me and he didn't tell me everything, but there's nothing you can do about it. He would tell me, but I just wouldn't know how serious everything really was. It's like I would be furious if they didn't tell me what was going on because I want to know what's going on with me, no matter what. I didn't want any surprises, I just wanted to know what was going on.

There were kids in the hospital that I would talk to, but they didn't have the same problem, they didn't have leukemia. They had different problems, different types of cancers. I didn't feel comfortable talking about it to other people because, like, one thing that I did realize through the whole thing was that you shouldn't really talk to other people with other problems about cancer because they'll get the wrong idea. I mean, I can remember my mom talking to different parents and listening to what the different parents were saying and stuff and it was terrible. And I would get all worked up over something that was a totally different type of cancer. You'd think it's, you know, it doesn't have anything to do with what you have. So you can't really go by what other people say, unless they have the exact same thing as you do.

And not even then because your body reacts totally different from everybody else's, everybody's body's different. It's a hard time and sometimes it gets harder than others, and sometimes it gets a lot less harder than others. I mean, it's just, it's the way your body reacts to the medications. You can never tell how it's going to work. It's worked out that my body worked out to this protocol. I mean, I know people here that have relapsed over and over, and I've gone straight through without any problems. It's been terrible. It's not fair. I hate that, I hate that. That's one of the things I hate the most, 'cause I don't understand why I went through it so good and they're still, they're getting, they're doing so terrible. They keep relapsing. One boy's been here since he's been I don't know how old, since he's been a baby and he still keeps relapsing. They still haven't found the right thing for him. I just don't understand how mine worked out so good and the other kids haven't.

I can't remember everything but there were times, the Cytoxan times, that were very hard times and my parents thought that I probably didn't want to go on and stuff. Thinking about it now even makes me cringe, not wanting to go through it again. I would not go through it again. I would not want to go through it again. But I know if I got it again, I would have to go through it again, and I would. I would go through it again until it goes away for good. But it's very scary, because I've been put back in place with everybody else again, and I feel totally normal right now and to have it put back on again would be terrible. I've got, I think, maybe a year and a half more left on the protocol. It's been I think about two years that I've been on treatment, and I've got one more year left and then I'll be in remission on this protocol and then I should be done with it.

There was a time when anything I asked for, people would jump to get it for me, I mean my family and stuff. But I wasn't realizing it, you know, you're not thinking about what people are doing for you and stuff while you're going through it, you only realize it afterwards. You seemed spoiled when everything's over with. Granted everything isn't over with for me. I still come in for some treatments, but it's not as intense as it used to be. And now that everything's over, most of the intense stuff is over, you feel that everyone's still gonna be jumping at any call you have. And yeah, I've noticed that I've been sort of spoiled with that, and it annoys people, but, like, they sometimes, then they'll stop and realize, you know, for a whole year, this kid's gotten whatever, anything he's wanted. So they've gotta accept it.

I mean one of the things that helped me get through was what my dad called "the Saturday prize." And what that was was every Saturday he would give me something to look forward to and I could get anything I wanted. And, you know, it helped a lot. It made me look forward to things, and it just kept coming and it made me look forward to the end. And then the end's here and now everything's fine.

My dad helps me in lots of other ways, like when I have to come here for the spinal taps. I mean, I couldn't do it without my dad. Because I'm big, a lot bigger than the other patients they've got here, and it's hard for them to get me in a tiny ball that they have to do for the spinal tap, and my dad always comes in and crinkles me into that ball. And he's there talking me through it all, because the spinal tap is the worst thing of all for me. And it's hard for the doctor to get to my back. But this doctor's a great doctor. He's definitely had a big uplift on it for me. And the nurses, I mean they were tremendous, they were great. Anything we wanted they would get, you know, they would be there.

I went back to school this year. This is my first year back to school. And, um, I started high school, freshman year but I didn't finish freshman year. I got diagnosed in the end of freshman year so they took me out of school. I didn't go back to school for my sophomore year. By the end of sophomore year, I was alright to be at home, and do everything at home, and even start school. I started home tutoring and the doctor kept saying, "Oh you can go back at Christmas," and then I didn't go back at Christmas, and it just went on and on and just ended up that I stayed the whole year of sophomore year out. All my friends knew was that, um, I had a cancer, but they didn't know what it was. They still don't know what it is, you know. But they know it was serious.

Most of the time I was out of school I didn't feel like seeing much of anybody. I didn't feel like anything. You don't want to be near anybody, you don't. It's sad but you can be rude to people and not know it. Because you're just out of everything. I hardly talked to them, even on the phone, except for towards the very end of the year, when I was getting a lot better. When I finally got back to school it was really good seeing all my friends again, yeah. During last summer I had seen a lot of my friends, but to see them all again, and to be back with everybody was a great feeling.

When I was going through it, I just felt so terrible. I didn't think I'd look good and I thought that I would just be, it's hard to say. It's so hard and so painful, some of the things are very painful. You get so sick you think you're never going to get better again. It's terrible. I couldn't see my friends. It wasn't really not wanting to see them, but not wanting them to see me, because I didn't feel good, and I didn't look good. I mean, you look terrible, your face bloats out. When I was going through it, I thought that, you know, that I was never going to be the same. But now I am. I mean I think I'm better now than I was before. Now I feel better than I did before I got sick because, you see, they said I could have had it since way back even 'til that Christmas before. So it could have been lingering in me for that long.

So I don't know, but I just feel like a whole new person now than I did before and all that. It made me stop and look at what's going on around me. I think that I'm taking things a lot more seriously, and I think that it was, um, a great, a really good experience for my knowledge, learning experience, and for my family's knowledge, a learning experience. And it just makes you have a lot of faith in the doctors and in what's going on. I know a lot more about cancer. I didn't let any of the doctors do anything to me unless I knew what they were doing and why they were doing it and what cause it was for. I mean, I always asked questions. And I probably know now more about leukemia than any of my teachers do or anybody else. I mean, it was a great learning experience.

I think it's helped me grow up more. I think that, um, yeah, it changed the way I look at things. It lets you put aside all the things, all the little things that aren't important, and not take what you have for granted.

If anybody had what I had, I'd tell them to just keep with the medication, and keep up hope because one day you'll be fine, hopefully, especially with the way the medicines are coming along now, these days. I mean, I feel like a totally normal person and I don't feel like, you know, none of my friends, I don't feel alienated at all. And nobody can tell that I had cancer. There will be rough times and it's gonna be very rough. But it ends, and the rough times goes away. There's only a very short period that it's going to be rough, maybe a couple months, and then slowly, it'll be fine.

Anyone who asks me about it, I tell them about it, I mean, I talk about it all the time. My friends are all curious of what was going on. They're always asking questions like, um, well, what was going on and I'll tell them about, say, the procedures that I go through and the things that I went through in the hospital. And, um, then they'll ask me what the procedures are for and I'll explain to them what each thing did for me. And they still don't understand, but they get an idea. Right now, one of my friend's mom has cancer and he's asked me to come and see his mom and I've talked to his mom and she's asked me questions. But I told her, you know, she has a different type of cancer than I do, so I don't know. All I can say is it's going to be rough.

Now, I feel totally comfortable about talking about it. I have no problem with it. Why shouldn't other people want to know about it, and why shouldn't I tell them if I know about it? I mean, why keep it, like, hush-hush when it's something I went through, I wanted to know all about it. I mean, so I would talk about it. Sometimes I like to talk about it. I mean I talk to the teachers about it, and they ask me questions and I tell them. I'm an authority on having cancer 'cause I had it, and I went through it, and now I can see what it does to people. And they ask me about it, and I tell them. Well, I mean the research has come so far, it should keep coming. They should keep working at it to make it even less a problem. And I mean the statistics from when a long time ago to now, the success rate has been amazing. And I mean, it's, I'm living proof of it.

And it's a great thing to see what these, the things the medication can do, is just amazing. You know, you can't understand how it works and how the doctors come up with the things just to help solve the problem of it all. It's amazing. You can't even start to wonder how they know it.

The best thing is to talk

to somebody

Well, it hasn't really bothered me, with the disease, you know. I just found out last week. I feel confident about it, about being in the hospital. Basically, I'm not worried about anything, you know. Like afterwards or right now, I'm not worried about anything. Like, I don't think anything negative will happen.

Well, I didn't find out until I came into here, but I was feeling sick, like two weeks before I came in, but I didn't think it was really serious. At the time when I came in, the night I came in to the hospital, I thought I'd be leaving that night. And then, you know, I found out I would be in here for so long. I was surprised. I really didn't know how serious it was. I thought cancer would be bad. I didn't know much about cancer. I thought cancer was like, bad, and I needed to be told that this kind of cancer could be curable and everything. I have Hodgkin's disease, with the lymph nodes being, I guess, enlarged, like all over my body. But after medication, it's curable. It was like, surprising to me, but after I knew it was curable, I felt a lot better.

It will take pretty long. They said like maybe eight months. So it will all be gone in maybe eight months. I'll have to take these medications, I don't know what they are called, but I'll have to take them like every two weeks, and then I'll have a two week break, and then I'll take it again, for like eight months, for an eight-month period. They told me that I can have fevers from it, high fevers a lot, and headaches, and I could feel nauseous a lot. And they told me, they tried to tell me what to do at home, if I'm at home, you know once I get out of the hospital. What to do, you know, when I feel like this. They said like I have to call the hospital immediately 'cause it could be just symptoms, but maybe it has to do with the disease.

They said it was just bad luck that it happened to me. I guess I understand that it has to happen, you know, to some people it just happens, bad luck. Just some things happen at the wrong time, I guess. Maybe I did something at the time that I shouldn't have done and that started the disease. They say that I couldn't have, that there was no way I could have avoided it. I don't think I could have avoided it. I don't think there's anything I did, like, you know, I don't think, like, I wasn't out in the rain, a cold rain or nothing like that, or improperly dressed. So I don't think I could have avoided it.

At first, when my mother was told about it, she was, I could see that she was very depressed. But then, as it went on and she found out that it was curable, she took it a lot easier. And thinking about my father and everything, you know. I mean, both of us being in the hospital at the same time and he's in a coma. It's like, unbelievable. He only went in a week before I did. But she takes it a lot easier now, you know, once she found out what it was, you know, that it was curable, she felt a lot easier about things.

I told my brother, but it's, like he's young, and I guess he doesn't think like the way older people would, you know, like he doesn't know what's going on. 'Cause he's young, eleven years old, so he doesn't know how to take it. If he were older maybe he would take it a lot harder. Like, he asked me, like, well, at first he asked me what I had, and everything, if I'll be all right. But now, like, he knows it's curable, and he's hoping that I get out soon and everything. I think now I've grown closer to him since I had it, you know. I talk to him more on the phone and everything. I just talk like how he's doing, and how I'm doing, and what he's doing around the house, and if he's doing what he should be doing.

I have one of my friends that came up to see me, and, well, he had already been told by his mother, 'cause my mother knows his mother. And he took it, you know, once he knew it was curable and everything, and by the time he saw me, he knew everything's all right and everything. And since it's curable, he asked a lot of questions like how I felt, and if it made me feel different than I was before, and everything. But, no, I feel the same. It's just my breathing is better now. I could breath a lot better and everything, 'cause before I couldn't, like if I walked upstairs, I'd be exhausted. But now I'm sure I'll be a lot better.

When I came to the hospital, I couldn't breathe, so they had to put me on the oxygen right away. That was scary. I was never in the hospital before, and I've never been to see anybody and, like, I never knew, I never knew what was going on. I didn't ask anything, I just stood there and took what was coming. You know when they put the oxygen on me real quick, I thought something was happening and everything. Well, I thought, you know, maybe I was close to dying. But my mom was there for me, and she had me calm and everything. I thought, you know, I just thought, things were going to turn out real bad, you know? When it happened, when it was happening, I thought, you know, like maybe after this, like, I wouldn't be able to talk, 'cause they did the biopsy on my neck. And I thought maybe I'd be hoarse or something like that. And it was really difficult to go through, you know, being awake. You could feel them like, cutting inside, you know, and like grinding into my throat and everything. And it was really horrifying. And that was late at night, it was like four o'clock in the morning, when they were doing it. The people were close and everything. They were saying all their hospital terms and everything and I could hear them. And when I don't know what's being said, I got scared. It was difficult to sit there and try to think what they're saying, you know, if it's bad or good, you know, while they were doing it. I thought something might have died in me and I might not come out of that.

I pray a lot, you know, at night and everything, that it'll help me through. I find it very helpful, at times. Well, now since I've been in the hospital, it's a lot of comfort. I do things, when I go to bed I do the same things, like read and other times, when I'm feeling like low, or something's going on in the hospital to me that's bad, you know, I'll do prayers from the book. Like, maybe if I was going for a biopsy, you know, and I knew about it, I'd like pray before the time, you know, from the book. I have a little religious book. I have it here, and it has different prayers in it.

You have to have a positive attitude, you know, towards, you know, what's going on. If you feel negative towards things, you'll be scared or something. But if you're positive, you'll feel good about things and it'll help you through like what you're going through. Like maybe if I feel positive, you know, maybe it wouldn't hurt as much, or maybe I'd get through it and feel a lot better going through it. Make sure you know, and you're thinking the best will happen. The best thing, like, is to be able to talk to someone. Like someone who can make you feel positive, you know, by talking to you and maybe know what's gonna happen. Like maybe if something's gonna happen to you that they'll be able to talk to you, make you feel like you know what's going on and you'll feel better about it. Like someone who's gone through it, that you know or something, like maybe another patient. And you know, they'll be able to help you a lot better than if you were just to talk to somebody that didn't know anything about it.

And if you're religious, you know, make sure you pray for yourself and pray for what's going on. And just try to be as positive, or if you're feeling low, you know, you gotta try to make yourself feel positive. The best thing is to talk to somebody. If you've got somebody to talk to, like a parent, or a patient, it's a lot easier. If there's something I don't know, I try to ask and get as much information out of it as I can. You know, and they try to stay away from hospital terms, and talk about it like so I would know.

Maybe if they told me things beforehand, because they don't really do it now. If they told me what was going on, what was gonna, like, if something was gonna happen, that I had to go for a biopsy or something, you know that they told me beforehand and made sure I was informed on everything that was gonna happen, it'd be better. Sometimes they don't tell you in enough time before or sometimes they don't inform you enough. They tell you late and it's not as much as you want to know. When I ask them, they go back to the same things they told me, you know, they don't, or sometimes if they know a lot they'll try to squeeze out just a little more information. But if they don't know, really know, or they don't know how to say it, they'll just go back to what they said. They just don't know what to say, you know?

Maybe they feel that there's some things they shouldn't have to tell me, or that they don't want to tell me, you know, 'cause it's too rough. Like, maybe I'll feel, like, really negative if they told me, you know. Like, if somebody went for a biopsy, if they expected just, like maybe just a little cut or something like that, and then they were really going for the throat, you know, maybe they wouldn't want to tell them. Maybe some persons, they just, if they had things told to them that are extreme like that, maybe they'll be scared. But I think it's better for me to know. And if, you know, if I know I've got to go through it, you know I'll just go through it.

Sometimes, you know, doctors try to do things as quick as they can, you know, and they think wisely, you know, the people that work, they work wisely. Hospitals are OK. I wouldn't suggest a long time in a hospital. Maybe by the time I get out of this hospital, I won't like it at all. I won't want to come back to a hospital.

I didn't feel myself

When you get the bone marrow, you have to stay in here for three months. It got boring; you couldn't go anywhere without a mask, and you couldn't go outside. I've been good for so many months, so I'm gonna get my broviac taken out and I'll be better. I was really really sick. I didn't feel myself. It makes your hair fall out and stuff, the chemo, and you have to stay in the hospital for like a month, and then you come out, but then you have to get in remission, then you go to get your bone marrow, and sometimes you can get the bone marrow from somebody else and sometimes you have to take your own.

I got it from my brother. It was like I thought I was gonna die, but he saved my life with the bone marrow. He was 8, when he gave it, and he just turned 9, and he even said that if I had to get it again, he'll give me more. But sometimes you're not lucky because you can't get a bone marrow from anybody and you have to get it from your own self, and I was a lucky because I got to get it from my brother. Most people can't get it, 'cause some people don't have brothers, and most people don't have matches. The other kids, they'll be good, too, and they'll get better. It was really scary. Maybe your kids won't get it.

The first days I came home for like two months, I couldn't have friends or anything, and I still can't have animals. I want to get two kittens, and one puppy, and my dog back. It was a springer spaniel named Daisy. We had to give her to my friend's house. I miss her a lot and I sent her a valentine card, that's what you can do, you can send her your favorite valentine's card, and my grandma died of cancer, too. I wish she could have died when I was not sick, because she could have hugged me better, because she couldn't hug me. After she died I couldn't hug her, and before she died I couldn't hug her. I thought I was gonna have a sickness and I was gonna die. It was like I wasn't going anywhere, it was just like I was gonna lay there all year long, every single year, and then one day somebody found me, laying there, Mommy and Daddy, and they buried me, and I miss everybody.

When you get sick, you don't feel good. When you have this kind of sick, you don't feel good, and I'm here now because I got a high temperature. If you get a high temperature, even if it's below really high, you can still go in the hospital. Cancer sickness you can't give to somebody, and mine came in my blood, and you can get it in a lot of other places. Cancer, like you have to stay in the hospital for five or six months and it's really dangerous because you can get sick. Because you can get a cold, and then you can get really a lot of germs, and then you might have to go in again, and sometimes, it's like you're at home, and you have to go in the hospital a lot of times.

You can play and talk to other people and try and forget it and stuff. You have to not think about it, you have to really play a lot, and when you play you can get it out of your mind when you're sick and you can pretend that you're at home. Some things you can't have when you want it, like your animals, like things you really want a lot. You can't have some foods and stuff, and some other things you can't have. Like if you want something special, you can't have it. Sometimes if you want something like an animal or food, you should try to get your mind off them and play some more and don't think about it.

The doctors have to make your blood better instead of bad blood, and I even had to get radiation to kill the other blood. It's stuff that makes your bad blood go away; it kills the germs. There's not kids around you. You have to stay home always, you never can go to school but you can go outside. I only went to school two times at nursery school, and after two days I got sick. I think after my birthday I'll be going to school, and before my birthday, I'm gonna get my broviac taken out, 'cause you have to get a broviac taken. I had to get a broviac because my blood veins weren't good, they couldn't get anything out of them anymore. It's the thing that you have in your chest and nobody can really see it, they put it in, and nobody really sees it.

For my sickness, I've been like eight or ten months, maybe even more, maybe twelve. Most of my friends aren't sick but I don't care because I know I'm gonna be better.

You're the only child in the world
that has it

Having cancer is really scary. I don't know how to describe it. Sometimes you think about it, you know, why it had to happen to you, things like that. You don't know what's going to happen to you if one day you gonna be on the street and something's gonna happen to you. At first, it was hard for me to sleep at night because I didn't know what was gonna happen, if I would wake up. Sometimes when I'm by myself, I think about what's gonna happen, am I gonna get better or get worse or, you know, what kind of changes your body is gonna go through, things like that.

When I first was told, I thought maybe if I go to sleep and wake up, I'll be dreaming. I wanted to know how could you get it because one day I was fine and the next thing I know someone's telling me I have leukemia. At first I just was in shock, I couldn't say anything about it, like that, but I don't really know how to explain it. You sit there, and when the doctor first told me, I looked at him like and I was waiting for him to tell me the rest, like it was a joke, and I sat there, and he tells me like, well, in two and a half years or so you'll be off medication, and I'm looking at him like, "Why does it have to be me? Why couldn't it be somebody else?" It felt like the end of the world, like, "Why did it have to happen to me, why me?" It's the question I always ask myself, even now. There is no answer. You think maybe you did something bad.

Another way that you feel when you first find out is that you're the only one who has it, you're the only child in the world that has it and nobody's gonna like you, everybody's gonna want to have nothing to do with you. But you have to think about the chance of you gettin' better, and then you try to cope with it, you try to accept it. Now I can sit there and I joke with him and it's not so bad after you get to know the doctor. I get medicine every day, and at first I couldn't eat certain things like I used to, like greasy food, like fried chicken, and I couldn't eat them at first because when I'd finish eating, I'd bring it back up. I lost a lot of weight. My hair started to fall out, and that's what made it worse, thinking, "I'm a girl, I need my hair." It didn't fall out all together, it just started to thin out. Then after a while, it grew back, and it grew back longer than it was before, and then it started to thin out again. Sometimes I look forward to coming to the doctor because he tells me, "Oh, you're getting better." I like to hear things like that, then I know I'm not supposed to give up.

I only told my family and two or three of my close friends and the rest, well, when I had left school last year everybody, well, I had a back tumor first, that's how I had found out, so everybody just thought I had to stay home the rest of the year because I had a back operation. One night I was with my best friend and we were just talking about what we did during Easter vacation. She just came back from visiting her family, and I started to tell her, "Remember when I was in the hospital, it was a little bit more than a back operation." And she sat down and she's like, "Stop playing," and I started telling her, and she started crying, and I'm sitting looking at her saying, "Why are you crying, I should be the one that's crying, it's me that's going through all of this." And she said, "No," because she didn't know what was going to happen to me either. She thought I was telling her that I'm dying or something like that. So we talked about it, and she told me whenever I don't feel well she'll help me. We'll sit there and talk, if I feel depressed or something like that. It draws us closer together, not further apart, because when I don't feel well it's like she doesn't feel well either, and if I'm crying, she cries.

Sometimes my other friends, like they baby me, and sometimes I feel, "Why did I tell you because now everybody wants to baby me," and everybody looks at me like, "How can you take it so well?" You have to accept it, you have to go on, if you give up that's the way I think you get even more sick. My mother tells me, if you give up and you give in, it just takes you over and that's it. That's saying, "I'm sick and I'm not going to get better." Like if I don't go to the doctor, if I don't take my medicine, it doesn't matter anyway, you know, because I might not get better, but I think, I know for sure I'm gonna get better. I still make plans, I try to be the same person I was before. If you let it change you in your attitude toward yourself, its just gonna take you over so that even when you're getting better, you're not gonna feel you're getting better because you're gonna have it in your head that "I'm not gonna get better."

At first I used to always make us late for our doctor's appointments 'cause I thought they're just telling me I'm gonna get better because that's what they want to make me feel. They just wanna make me smile. At first I didn't trust anyone, even my mother. She used to tell me, "You're gonna get better," and I'd say, "Yeah, I'm gonna get better," but when she would turn her back I'd say she's just telling me that because I'm her daughter, she's supposed to tell me that, not because it's really true. But if my doctor wanted to talk to her separately, I'd say, "No, I want to listen, I want to hear every detail," and the doctor looked at me like, "We're not hiding anything." "Well, if you're not hiding anything then why can't I listen?" And I'd say, "I'd rather know everything, so I'd rather you talk to me than you talking to my mother because I think I'm old enough to understand because I'm the one that's gonna go through all of this." And now everything is getting better. I started talking to the doctor, and I asked him, "Am I really gonna get better?" And he said, "Yeah, in two years or so, you won't be coming to see me anymore," and things like that. And I'm looking forward to that. I mean, I like my doctor now, but I'm looking forward to when I won't have to come here.

You have to talk to your doctor so you can understand, so if he says something's wrong, like your progress is slowing down, you have to know. You can't hear it from your mother because your mother might be scared to tell you that. You have to hear it for yourself. Maybe you're thinking, I'm not taking my medicine like I should, maybe I'm not getting enough rest or things like that. When I first started coming here I didn't talk to anybody. When he would say he was going to examine me, I'd say, "What is this, what is that for?" And he'd say, "You don't trust me?" and I'd say, "Well, to tell you the truth, I don't trust anybody," because they gonna think that because I'm a child, I'm not gonna understand. Then slowly, as he started telling me, he said, "I'm telling you the truth, you're gonna get better." I look at my chart that tells how long it will take for the process, it says what each medicine does, things like that. Then slowly I started thinking he knows what he's talking about, he knows what he's doing, so I started to trust him little by little. I asked him a lot of questions, and he likes that when I ask him questions because that makes him think, that gives me an advantage. That makes him think, "Oh, she's on top of me, she's asking me questions."

If you talk to somebody, don't keep it all inside, you can't deal with it on your own, and don't feel sorry for yourself, that's another thing. If you give in, and say, "Well I might die anyway," you can't think like that because that's not true, because when I first heard about it, every time I heard on the news about somebody having leukemia, I always thought, "Well they're going to die, they're not gonna get better." That's why I cried a lot at first, and in a way that's good if you feel depressed to cry. That helps you deal with it in your own way. At first, I was sitting here and I cried and I cried, and my mother and my father were telling me that it was going to be OK, but then my father said to my mother to let me cry because that was the way I could deal with it.

I talk to my father and tell him how I feel, like maybe sometimes I feel like giving up, and he tells me, "No, you can't do that, you can't give up, darling, you can't do that." Everybody in my family tells me that I'm a strong person, if I have my mind set on something, I always go and do it no matter what anybody says or thinks. Just don't give up. When that happens, you just don't care anymore, you don't ask any questions, you just come to the doctor and he gives you the medicine, and you just go home, you don't ask anything, you don't talk about it, things like that.

My family's got a lot closer because of this. Like we all got closer together because when everybody has their own time, they wanted to be alone, like in their own little moods and sometimes I get my little moods, and I say, "Leave me alone, I don't feel like talking." But my sisters would keep bothering me, "Why you don't feel like talking? You want to go shopping, you want to go to the store with me?" They'll keep asking me, they don't like me to sit there with a sad look on my face because that makes them think I'm probably thinking something is wrong so, "Let's not leave her by herself because I don't want her to sit there and get depressed." So it brought us closer together, but they still treat me the same—we still argue, we still fight, we still argue over the telephone, about clothes, money, the bathroom. Everything is still the same. When I came home from the hospital I told them, "I'm the same person I was before I went to the hospital, so don't treat me any differently."

Most of the time when I get depressed, I think about my mother cause she has to deal with all of this, all of this is on her mind. Like sometimes I go into her room and she'll be crying or something like that, and I ask her why she's crying, "I'm not crying, something's in my eye," or something like that because she thinks about how I'm reacting because I'm so young and how I'm dealing with all of it. At first, I was more depressed than I am now. I never wanted to get dressed, I never wanted to leave the house, I would stay in front of the TV, wake up and go to sleep, my appetite wasn't that good. But now that I went back to school, I like everything about my home life, I'm on the phone, or I'm going out with my friends.

I'm gonna get better and then I would think about how I overcame my obstacles, a big obstacle in my life. So if something else like this ever would come up again, then I know I could do it because I've done it before. When I'm older, that will make me think that I'll have a better chance, everything to me will be brighter because I faced something that not a lot of people can overcome. So anything that comes my way, any obstacle that comes, I can overcome it because I did it once before.

Common narrative themes

Each child with cancer experiences it in his or her own way, and expresses that experience in a unique voice. Yet almost all of the children at some point in their stories spontaneously bring up issues that reflect common themes about their struggle to cope with having cancer. These themes are: "Why me?"; the role of God and prayer; fears about having cancer; losing their hair; advice for others who have cancer; how having cancer tests friendships and family affiliations; how having cancer has changed their attitudes and social behavior beyond the context of cancer; and talking about talking about cancer.

Why me?

Soon after coming to understand the implications of a cancer diagnosis, almost every child questions why this is happening to him or her. Children who do not pose this question to themselves are denying, to varying extent, the emotional impact of having cancer.

The question "Why me?" has no answer. How children resolve this question, therefore, is a projection of their struggle to attribute meaning to an emotionally painful and seemingly arbitrary series of circumstances. It is also a prognostic indicator of children's ability to emotionally adjust to the continuing uncertainties of treatment. Children who are unable to resolve the question "Why me?" in their own way are not able to accept the vicissitudes of treatment and continually resist it as something that is inherently unfair.

Resolution of this question comes in a variety of forms. Some children attribute their illness to the will of God and accept that, as God is the source of their distress, their faith and prayer will be their road to recovery. Other children resolve it in terms of one of many uncertainties and chances in life that somehow are randomly distributed among the population. Some children come to justify their cancer as a form of punishment; and, of course, children always can find something that they had said or done that was morally culpable and worthy of punishment. But for many children it is particularly difficult to reconcile why they suffer when others who obviously are more blameworthy, such as criminals, remain free of disease.

A few children attribute rational causality when there is no evidence to support it, such as cancer being caused by their diet or environment. However, the propensity to attribute rational causality to a child's cancer is not as common among children as it is among their parents. I once asked twenty mothers about this and seventeen of them gave me their reasons why their children had cancer. They typically were attributed to emotional strife and stress within the family environment, such as marital discord, the loss of a member of the family, or financial problems. The attending physician of each child had assured me that he or she personally had advised the mother that there was no known scientific cause for her child's cancer, and although about half of the mothers clearly recalled being told this, they were still confident that they knew the cause as it pertained to their particular child. The other mothers did not remember being so advised by their physician, but they also showed no inclination to test their attribution of causality against their physician's opinion. The need to find a reason why their child has cancer reflects the parents' overwhelming fear and unwillingness to accept the unknown, particularly when the consequences are so devastating and life-threatening. In considering causes of childhood cancer, it is interesting to note that the idea of a cancer-prone personality type is an attribution that adults often inflict upon themselves and others as a cause of cancer, but never upon their own children.

Children seem better able to resolve the "Why me?" question than their parents and, consequently, are better able to adjust to this initial phase of the cancer experience. Children often recognize this difference between themselves and their parents and express it in terms of how learning about their cancer was tougher on their parents than on themselves.

The following are some of the ways in which children approach and attempt to resolve the question "Why me?":

———————

You always say "Why me?" but you didn't do anything to deserve it, no one does anything to deserve it, it's just something that happens, so you can't say "Why me?" It could happen to anyone, but it happened to you, so maybe the big guy upstairs wanted it to happen to you to make you an example to everyone else that you can battle it, and show that you can make it. You didn't do anything, you didn't not eat your vegetables, so you got cancer, you didn't go out and kill a squirrel so that's why you got cancer, you didn't do anything that you can get it from, or not do anything, it just happens.

———————

I felt I was being punished, and I thought that I had done something really terrible and this is God's way of punishing me, and then I realized, my mother made me see, that it doesn't happen to everybody, and it doesn't happen to the good people or the bad, it just happens, not because it was meant to be, but because there's something with your body inside.

———————

The first couple of days, I used to cry sometimes, I still do sometimes when I get pain in my arms from the medicine reaction, and you start thinking, "Why me? Why don't criminals get sick, why don't bad people get sick, politicians, why me?" and you start telling God, "I haven't done nothing bad to deserve it," and you just have to accept it and be strong cause if you don't accept it and be strong, you gonna let the sickness get to you.

———————

This semester everything was going well, and I used to tell people, "Something bad is going to happen to me," and now I got leukemia, things were too good.

I mean, people sometimes think that they did something, and that made them get cancer. Oh, Mom said not to get drunk and I got drunk, so I got cancer from that. No. You did nothing and nobody did anything to or toward you. I mean, and you didn't do anything toward anybody to get it. You just got it. And that's that. You know, that's one thing that a lot of people should learn. You didn't do anything to get it.

I was just thinking "Why me?" I thought, why couldn't it be somebody that does wrong, or somebody that does crime, or somebody that doesn't live right. And I thought that I don't see why I caught it. I thought it was from like, not um, taking care of myself. I thought it would be something like, 'cause of something that I ate. But then, I thought, I said, that, well, like they say, people catch stuff not because sometimes they, um, they just catch it. I kept thinking that I caught it 'cause I be around people that smoke, and you see the smoke goes in your face. I thought, I'm inhaling it, and that it caused me to get cancer. But sometimes I just think, it always gotta be a reason why you caught something. It always gotta be a reason cause nobody just catch nothing, something for nothing.

I got a twin brother, and I say, "Why did it happen to me and not him or my other brother?" I guess I just came out to be the one with the bad luck in the family. After a while I realize it just comes and goes. You just wonder why God wanted us to be like this.

I thought "Why me?" because, it's like, I didn't do nothing wrong, I didn't do a crime or drugs or smoke or drink, and it happened to me. And I'm just like a kid, who stays away from the society of bad influences. And I get caught with a big problem, and they have a better life. I don't know what to think because it happened, it happened, you know. But it's frustrating like, you don't know how it happened. 'Cause it could be pollution, cancer could be what you ate. I don't know. Um, me, I see it like, 'cause I didn't like to eat, like, it's not that I like junk food, it's just that I didn't like to eat. So I got skinny. And probably since that it was in the bone, the cancer, probably a lack of nutrients to go to the bone, probably caused cancer. That's the way I see it. I don't know.

That's probably the reason why I'm here now, because of me messing with somebody that I shouldn't have been bothering, you know. It probably just came back to me, like they say, what goes around comes around. It probably just came around to me. Like, whatever caused the tumor, whatever, it all boils down to one thing, I got punished for something I shouldn't have been doing. And that's probably part of the punishment. It's just coming all down in one ball, you now, something like that.

Sometimes I think that, "Why do I have this disease?" But, um, you know, when I talk with my parents, or my grandparents, or whoever, I tell them, "Why do I have this?" And my father said God gave it to me, "God is the one that gave you this. This is life. Life gives you some tough punches and you have to face them." And I think, sometimes I think, but there's people that have it worse. They have worse problems. So I think to myself I'm not the only one and there's people that have worse problems than I have.

———————

Why did this happen to me? Before the cancer, I was healthy, nothing was wrong with me. I had my hearing and my eyesight was okay. Then this happened. Why me? I kept asking the doctors that. They gave me bullshit, telling me that people get a tumor, it just happens.

God and prayer

Often, in order to help resolve the question "Why me?" children turn to God and prayer. For many children, whether they come from religious families or not, faith in God becomes an important way of dealing with the pain, frustrations, and side effects of treatment. When they are trying to come to grips with the fear of dying and, sometimes, with the inevitability of impending death, many children find solace in putting themselves in the hands of God.

I think it's been different for me than for a lot of other people because my belief in God is strong, and I did go through the thing of the feeling of sadness and all of that, yet I was still, I was always in the Church, and there was always people there encouraging me to keep me going, and I feel like my religion has really kept me up. I feel so different because of my belief in God and it keeps me going strong. I have something to depend on, to believe that it will be over.

I know I'm gonna get cured because I have faith in God. I used to pray even before I had cancer every night and now I do an extra prayer, after my regular prayer at night, I pray a little bit more. I talk to God, tell him how I feel, tell him to try to help me out, get more through every day, day by day help me get through this. Cancer really doesn't do nothing to my mind that much, only at night time when I talk to God about it.

God's gonna cure you, second come the doctors they cure you with the medicine, first God and with the doctors' help and with God's faith you're gonna beat it out. If you don't beat it, that means God needs you up there. There's nothing you can really do about it, you have leukemia. I'm not gonna kill myself just because I have leukemia. You gotta enjoy life, enjoy all the little things you enjoyed before you had leukemia and give more than you did before, do more of God's work than you did before.

I said to my teacher, I wish God gave me cancer, so I could prove to everybody that I could beat it, and now I got it. I'm not sure I really wanted it, I just said it playing around. Now I really believe in God because I used to tell God I want cancer, so I can be real famous when I make it in baseball, and tell people that I had it, and I could beat it. And I have it now, and now I have to really prove to God. Maybe He gave it to me to tell me if you really want it, you have it. It was weird.

. . . that made me feel good, 'cause a lot of the nurses were like, "Good luck, I'm praying for you," and I was praying for myself too. I couldn't worry, after praying I don't worry.

You pray and whatever happens, happens, and you pray for your family, if something happens to me, let them stay strong.

I know that once I pray, that it'll make a big difference cause I know something good is going to come out of whatever I'm praying for. Like if I'm praying that Russia might get rid of their bombs, I know something good will come, they probably will get rid of their bombs and become friends with the United States for a long time. I know that something good comes out of praying. So that's why I give it a chance to pray.

Well, lately I've been reading the Bible, which is something I should have been reading a long time ago, but it, it was just put off. And it's surprising, all the little details in it that I didn't know. And stories that are commonly known, but commonly known incorrectly. I've been reading it partly as a piece of literature, but I'm keeping my eye open for the inspirational part. I'm not sure what I believe in right now, and it's, I hope it will help me figure out what I do believe.

I think of God when I'm in trouble. At home I pray a lot, every night I pray. Here I just look up and ask God to help me fight this disease. I basically ask him to help me with this disease. I go to church and I believe that he can cure.

Before I had cancer they were talking about a bone tumor and I was praying a lot. And then when I found out I had cancer, like I started to slack it off. I still pray though, now and then.

Fears about having cancer

There are hardly any experiences that we can imagine that are more frightening for a child than to have cancer. It is a terrifying disease. The treatments are painful, and the uncertainty of whether a child will live or die is unremitting. Thus, we expect children to be afraid of having cancer and to express their fears of pain and suffering, of being different and isolated in the eyes of their peers, of losing parts of their body, of not achieving remission, of relapse, and of death and dying. Children who do not express any of these fears either are denying them or are facing their fears alone, without the support and comfort of others.

Listening to children talk about these kinds of fears is particularly difficult and painful for adults because they amplify our own fears. They go to the very heart of what we want to protect children from, and listening to them exposes our inability to protect them. Thinking that we can protect children, and unconsciously trying to protect ourselves, we sometimes unwittingly deny children the opportunity to talk about their fears about having cancer. By trying to reassure children that conditions are not as morbid as they might seem, we discourage them from acknowledging their fears and targeting them in appropriate ways.

As soon as children begin to tell us how afraid they are, it is not uncommon for adults to tell them, "There's nothing to worry about, everything will be all right," or "Don't dwell on the bad things, just think about the good things." These kinds of messages convey to children that adults do not want to hear about their fears, that it is inappropriate to talk about them, and that there is something wrong with them if they are not able to deny these feelings. However, no amount of denial will reduce the pain of chemotherapy, radiation treatments, spinal taps, or bone-marrow aspirations. Therefore, it is essential that these children know that anyone would be afraid of these procedures and that such fears are reality-based. As they become more familiar with the effects of these procedures, their fears will be reduced, even though the pain may remain.

Of all the fears associated with having cancer, fears of death and dying are the most difficult for us to accept, and so they are more likely to be expressed indirectly by children in the form of dreams, play, innuendos, and slips of the tongue. Yet it is impossible to hide the knowledge that other children in the hospital who have cancer are dying and that the conditions of the children who are dying in many cases are very similar to the conditions of those who are surviving. Children become close friends with other children in the hospital who have cancer, and they share their most intimate thoughts and feelings. In many cases it is easier for children who have cancer to be intimate with a peer who has cancer than with anyone else.

When they see that friend dying, the effects can be emotionally devastating. They must deal with their grief and mourning over the loss of their friend while simultaneously facing renewed fears about the possibility of their own death. Under these circumstances, the children's fears of dying need to be accepted while they can be comforted with knowledge that the treatment teams are doing everything they can to help them, to cure them.

The following are some of the ways in which children talk about their fears of having cancer:

———————

I never thought about dying. I feel good right now, you know. And I feel strong. And I never think about dying, I just think about, sometimes I think about if the cancer comes back, what I'm going to do. And I don't think I'm going to be able to handle it because of that. I'll just probably go crazy or something. I don't think I'll accept it, you know. Like after you fight so much, then it comes back all the time. And you gotta start another fight again. It just, well I just can't handle that and there's no way to know when it'll happen. The doctors don't even know.

———————

I thought, like, when you get cancer you die because I just see like old people and when they have cancer, they die, so I was thinking, "Dag, what if I die." And then I found out that some people get chemo treatment and you can still die from cancer, so that blew me out right there, that for a while couldn't put that down. I was thinking, I just wanted to tell them, "You gave me chemo, and I could still die?" I just wanted to tell 'em, and I didn't know how. I just wanted to tell the doctor, like well, "Don't you know you're giving me chemo treatment and I could still die from cancer, that don't mean nothing."

———————

I got scared when they said, "malignant tumor," so if they meant the same thing as cancer, then I guess I was just wondering why they didn't call it cancer. It was like, is it or is it not a different thing? That's what I was wondering and I got really scared. It's, just like, lonely scaredness, like nobody else knows how you feel.

It's not like you can't die from this because you can die, so you always think of death, but I don't think of it as anything that could happen because I'm doing so well. Once in a while when things aren't going well, you just think about, "Well, all of this is gonna go bad, and then you gonna die," but it doesn't happen that way, and it won't.

So my mother picked me up from school and she took me to the doctor and she told my mother it was a tumor. But I didn't know what it was, a tumor. So my mother started crying, and I knew that something was wrong. So I went home and looked in the dictionary, and I looked up for tumors, and they said it was a disease, that you could die. Then I got real scared, it scared me a lot. I was scared that I was going to, like, die. I was thinking about the tumor and I thought I was going to die. I started having dreams about these people chasing me and I went through this alley and I couldn't go out. And I started waking up sweaty.

It's scary because it's a potentially fatal dose of chemo that they're gonna give ya. But it's also, it's just not wanting to go back to the hospital, is more like it. I know what I'm in for.

You know, I dread it something fierce. But it has to be done, it will be done, and hopefully it'll be over as soon as possible.

I was really scared. One, I was very small and, two, it was my first time going to a hospital. And since when I was very little I used to watch a lot of TV and I used to hear about hospitals and needles and stuff like that. And the minute I heard, the minute I heard like that I was going to have to be taken to the hospital, I just really freaked out. I remember like my father had to carry me there and I was just crying and crying 'cause I was like really scared. I was just scared about the whole bit. I'm saying it's really scary. All these needles and poking. I mean, like I remember in the hospital from all the needles they used to give me my arms used to get black and blue all over. You know what's funny, well, my mother, we've been talking about this, we've talked about it. And my mother said the reason why she didn't tell me some things is because like she thought I might get really scared and worried.

It's sad and it's scary, 'cause I thought that I was going to lose my leg. If they wanted to put a prosthesis in it 'cause they was gonna take it off 'cause they said the tumor was like going to the bone, then they'd have to take the whole leg off. Well, I thought I was going to lose my leg. In a way I thought I was going to die too 'cause, like, I felt that if they took the leg off, then I couldn't be, I had to use a crutch, and I was thinking, what if the cancer would have spreaded, before they took off the leg, then I thought, it would probably came back after I got off the chemo. But then the doctors, after one of my friends passed away, they asked me if I was scared, did I worry about, like, the cancer coming back? I told them, "No."

If you find out you're gonna die, of course, it's a problem. Then you ask why this is happening to you, or why you're gonna die. Like, once you understand that, like say if this is a disease and sometimes there's not a cure for the disease that you have, then you don't understand why, why you're gonna die. But some of the doctors, they'll tell you that they'll try their best.

Now, I've gotta walk around now, thinking, and when I do get off the treatment, I gotta walk around thinking, I hope it don't come back. I gotta wonder if it's gonna come back or not. Like, day after day, that's the only thing that'll be affecting my mind. I know it. I know every day I'm gonna be running to the doctor, every day to find out if it came back or not. 'Cause I'm gonna be scared then. I'm gonna be more scared than I am now. 'Cause now I ain't worried about nothing 'cause I'm on the treatment. But when I get off the treatment, I'll be scared again. 'Cause I'll be like wondering, is it gonna come back or not.

One time I stayed in the hospital like two months, maybe more than two months, and I was very sick and I had a big fever, 106. I was very sick and I slept on ice bags and one night they wouldn't let me sleep because they were scared, scared that when I sleep I wouldn't wake up.

I haven't really gone that deep into it, but what I have done, I don't know, it's kind of hard to explain. You know, you think of what's going to happen, what could happen to you. And you know it's not, uh, fun, it's not a joyous occasion. Um, to think about that there's a possibility that you could die. Somewhere along the line if something went wrong. Um, and that's really all, you know, the possibility that I could die, that's the only thing that really bothers me, you know. I just, I really don't dwell on it that much. I just sort of look at what the results have been so far and what the doctor says. You know, that it's not that I'm going to die but this thing, this thing, I can't say it but you know, the chance, you know, death has crossed my mind at different times, but it's hard to explain it.

I don't really know, they haven't gone into long-term effects with radiation. As far as I know, there really are no long-term effects but it's always worrying me, I mean, it's always on my mind. I mean, uh, you always hear how, I was watching the news last night, and they said that how many x-rays you should get on your teeth, at the dentist, a year, because of the radiation. And you just think, x-rays on your teeth are like, you know, a quick snap. And this radiation's going on for 25 seconds, on each side, the machine flips around, and it does top and bottom. And it's always made me wonder, um, why on TV they're saying a quick x-ray, you know, how many times per year. And with this, they're not really going into the details, they're only saying that it might effect me while it's going on.

A lot of people, about three people I had made friends with, passed away while I was still on treatment. It was very upsetting. Because you know, it could have been me. Am I next?

I always get nervous when I come in for check-ups that they're going to find something. But, um, I'm just hoping that it doesn't come back. It seems like a very long time ago. I mean four years is a long time, but you always think about it.

———————————

So when I heard it I was like, that's when I started crying. I was really scared, it was worse than dying to me. I thought like, since it got fractured I thought I'd get my arm amputated. I just couldn't take that.

———————————

I had to ask myself that week how would I tolerate it if I'm told I might die, and now I've made some resolutions. I've thought about it more seriously than the fantastic way you think about it when you're just a little kid lying in bed saying, "Gee, what would happen if I died right now," so that week that I didn't know if I was going to make it, I had to actually come to terms with it. I managed to say, "OK, I've had a pretty good life so far." I mean I'm gonna die at some point, what's going to keep me going, it's going to be that I hope that I can have some influence on the people who are still alive, like my brother, my sister, and maybe they can pass part of what I've influenced in them to the people they see, and it will just go on geometrically. Those are the things that are important to me so I look back and I think have I had any influence, and I told my father this and he said, "Don't worry, you've had influence on people," so then I realized at that point that if I did have to go it wouldn't be that I did absolutely nothing, that it wasn't all for nothing.

I've also thought about the process, it's not going to be bad dying, it's going to be bad the couple hours before, the days before, after I'm dead it's OK. I've pretty much come to the conclusion that after you're dead you're gone and you don't think about anything, that wasn't what I was fearing. I was fearing the hours before, the days before, the unknown. But the thing that always got to me at the end is that I'm so young, it's not long enough a life, there's still so much to do, and if people tell me I'm so nice to them, then I have to do more with it, I can't stop now, I haven't had a family, kids.

Um, I was, um, I felt lucky that it wasn't me. Because like me and him was the same age. And I thought like, well, he shouldn't have got cancer, but I felt like maybe he should have got it when he was old. 'Cause he ain't lived no life. I thought, um, like he was, I knew he was sick, but I thought like he would hold on for like maybe two or three more months, because he didn't look, like, sick. He was talking to me, and he offered us some gum, and he was laughing with us. But like, two weeks later, he died. Um, well, I knew that I'm not going to die, I just, you know, just feel funny, 'cause, you know, 'cause when I first met him, you know, he was well, he was active. And it's hard to imagine that he's gone now. His chemo didn't help.

It's kind of hard, just seeing your friend, you know, and knowing that he ain't gonna make it. It's pretty hard even though I pretty much knew he ain't gonna make it. He had told me a week before he wasn't doing good. And he had told me that same day that he wasn't doing good, so I kind of knew. I was expecting it. The last time I saw him he just talked about everything we used to talk about, like sports, and basketball, activities like that. He wouldn't have talked about dying. Only with Danny, I think, 'cause Danny asked. I know Danny wanted to talk to him about it.

I mean, everybody was, I mean nobody was really shocked, but everybody was still hurt. Even though we knew it was gonna happen, we didn't want it to happen this fast. We was hoping that he would stay alive two more months at least, so we could at least see and talk to him. Everybody was hoping like the same. Everybody was saying at least two more months or so, so you could at least get to see him, if you come to the hospital, and you're a patient here, in-patient, and you could talk to him or something. No one was really shocked but it still hurt. 'Cause nobody had died before that. But then Steven died, and two weeks later he died, so people handled it better. The second time around it could work both ways, because somebody might just get mad and say, "Two guys died," and say, and you start saying something, like, "Are you gonna be next?"

It makes me mad to see one of my friends is dying, and I don't like to see one of my friends dying 'cause one moment they enjoying themself with me and the other guys, and the second moment they in bed, thinking about death, and that hurts, seeing them like that. 'Cause I see some of my friends, I know that even though the disease they got is tough on them, they really know that when they going to die, they take it slow, take it one day at a time. They don't want to get all panicky, not the friends that I know of. Like, get all hyper, I'm gonna die, and a lot of people say that if I were gonna die, I'd go crazy, I'd do this. See, most of the people I know, like if they knew they were going to die, they wouldn't get panicky, they'll probably start praying, just taking it one day at a time.

When I went into my friend's room, we was, all three of us, we was talking about, um, how he was doing, and stuff like that. And we was just talking about the basketball game, talking about things like that. But then, I asked them to leave for a moment 'cause I wanted to talk to him alone. And then when they left, he asked me what's the matter. I told him I couldn't see him like that. I couldn't see one of my friends all sick and dying. And what's wrong with us and everything. I said I'd rather see him out there with us enjoying himself, like the rest of us was. Then he said he knew how I feel, 'cause all the times when I had a headache, or I had a fever, and he came in my room, and he kept going back and forth out the room, he didn't want to see me like that. So he said he understands.

I was close to him because of the fact of what he had, leukemia, for me seeing what he was going through was a real bad thing, you know, 'cause he stayed in bed and he stayed sick, and one day he just pops up out of bed like nothing's wrong with him or nothing. They let him go home for a while, then he comes back sick again, and then a couple of days later he's dead, like that quick. Some people have and some people don't. It's bad, it hurts, 'cause you think that could happen to me too, you know then again it may not happen. In this hospital you go through a lot, it's hard to look at somebody that's dying and have to talk to him. I can't handle it.

It'll be like I'm gonna live my normal life like I always lived. Once again, like that. Have my hair back and be a normal person, just like I never had it. It's just that I'll always be thinking, if it's going to come back or not one day. That's the only thing.

Losing your hair

Compared with issues of death and dying, losing one's hair—an almost universal side effect of chemotherapy—does not seem so important to an adult. But it must be very important for these children, because almost all of them talk about what it is like for them to lose their hair and to have to cope with their baldness, if only temporarily during the course of their chemotherapy.

The loss of hair represents a particular phase in the progression of cancer. Upon first entering treatment, children see other children with cancer who have no hair and they feel different from them. Even when told that they too will lose their hair, they still feel separate from these bald children. Some children cling to the hope that others lose their hair but that it will not happen to them, and in rare cases that can be true. But almost always the loss of hair is the badge of cancer, and when it happens, children publicly enter the world of cancer. They can no longer pretend to themselves or try to hide from others that they have cancer.

It's scary. They tell you right from the beginning that you're going to lose your hair and you're constantly reminded of it, you know it's going to fall out, you keep meeting patients who

haven't got any. With me at least, I was amazed at how fast it
fell out. Suddenly, it started. For about two or three weeks, I
didn't lose any hair at all, but I knew it would be coming, but
that it takes a while, and then, one day in the shower, wash-
ing my hair, I looked at my hands, and it's amazing how much
hair falls out at once. And you've been expecting it for the last
couple weeks but it's still a shock. And in a couple of days, it's
noticeable. And that's a shock, too. And then, say, within five
days, it's down to having this much hair. Practically none.

And it was also surprising that it stopped falling out. I was
told that this will probably fall out in a little while, too. The
medicines I'm receiving, these ones are different from the ones
I received the first time, so I kind of expected that they might
cause more hair loss, or even if they were the same they might.
And it's difficult. If I were older, I don't think I'd particularly
care. I might be able to handle it better, but it's still scary to
everybody. And it takes a while to get used to what you look
like. Today is the first day I went out without wearing a hat. I
thought I'd try it for a while. And it hasn't been too bad, really.

I started getting really sad, and I started pulling my hair out,
one bit by bit, and my mom saw me pulling my hair out so she
called up the, um, the haircut person and then that's when he
started cutting my hair. This man came over to my house, I
had to go in the kitchen, and, um, I sat on a chair and he had
to cut all my hair, and I was bald. That really was bad. I didn't
want my hair to fall out. I didn't really like it.

Last week, when I came to the clinic, it was the first time I've
been in public with any hair loss. And I wore a hat. And I still

felt uncomfortable. And I got really nervous, I wasn't sure why. I thought it had to be something with that, I'm not completely sure it was that, either. And, if you're not happy with the way you look yourself, you think you must look strange to other people.

Deciding what to do about your hair loss is a whole problem in itself. Because last Friday I guess, my mother and I went to see about getting a wig. And even talking about that was hard. Because I just felt uncomfortable talking about it with my mother. And she knew I felt uncomfortable so she didn't talk about it. And I think she realized that I probably wanted one so people won't stare at me. I tried some on and I realized that I didn't like it at all. For some people, if they like it it's OK, but I felt very uncomfortable with it. So I decided against it. And then that night we went out to dinner. And I felt strange in a restaurant with my hat on, because I felt like I should take my hat off, but I knew I'd feel even more uncomfortable if I did.

I would guess people would think that something medical caused it to happen, like it was a fire and it burned off, or it could be a number of things. But they certainly would think something, 'cause your hair, your head is where your hair was. So it's obvious that there was hair there once. So they know something strange caused you to lose your hair. But also the fact that it just looks different. Just as if I came in with green hair, it would look just as strange. And it takes a while to get used to it yourself. I think once you get used to it yourself, it's easier to feel like other people won't be staring so much.

The strangest thing is seeing the back of your head behind your ear, 'cause it's always covered with hair. I've never seen that before. And even the way the hair sits a little differently after ninety percent of it falls out. My hair was a little long before it started falling out and I needed a haircut actually. But I decided not to get one 'cause it was going to fall out anyway.

And that was a mistake, for one thing. For anybody who's gonna have their hair fall out, I'd say get it cut short. Because it's very messy when it falls out because you don't realize how much hair you've got until you're pulling it out every day.

I'm starting to get comfortable with it. But that's another point that a lot of people are afraid to talk about. And with me, I was able to joke about that, too. And I think that helps. Other people will be able to do so also, but they'd still be careful. And honestly, I'd like them to be careful. I don't want people just, all day, you know, talking about my hair.

Another strange thing about it, that I wouldn't expect, is the way it falls out. You don't just get a bald spot and it spreads, or a receding hairline. It doesn't really fall out in clumps. But certain areas will fall out faster than others. Although overall, eventually it seems to even out. But the right side of my head fell out much faster than the left side. Luckily I part my hair on the left, so it sweeps to the right, and it covered it and made it look sort of even. But around the ears it fell out much faster. And I've always liked my hair to come down to my ear. And seeing the head above my ear has never appealed to me. So it took me a while to get used to. But once it's all out, that's the image I have of having cancer. That it makes you feel like your whole body is decaying.

I can go to school, but I don't want to 'cause I don't have no hair, and everybody in there got their nice haircuts, and I go in there and I don't have no haircut, I have nothing at all. I have to wear a hat, and then some teacher will be like, "Why you got the hat on?" and I got to explain to them why I got my hat on. And then my friends, all of them got their nice different haircuts, and I gotta wear a hat all the time. If they do things, I do whatever I could to avoid the fact that I gotta take off my hat.

Like when I go skating, you gotta take your hat off when you go skating and I'd be like, God, I can't even get on the floor because I got a bald head. And I wasn't going to go out there looking different from everybody else. Everybody else got all these different haircuts and I gotta go out there with no hair at all? You know, that there'd be some people who'd be, like, just forget what other people say, forget what other people say, that's you. But I feel like this, I don't want to go out there, 'cause if I go out there, everybody'd start looking at me, just me. Everybody'd look at me like I was a certain individual, like, and some of them might laugh, and some of them might feel bad, 'cause some people probably understand what it is. So I just, you know, I don't go skating, I just sit around, you know. And I won't even go to school now because of that. You see, 'cause I could go to school, but I don't want to go to school and be sitting in a class, sitting there with no hair, and everybody got hair. And everybody just sitting around talking about you, all the little groups talking about you, and you sitting there by yourself looking like a dummy.

Sometimes, I feel funny walking up to a girl and saying, "How you doing?" and they be like, "Take your hat off for a minute." And I'm like, "No." And they say, "Why not?" and I'm like, "'Cause I don't wanna," and they be like, "I just wanna see your haircut," and I be like, "You can't see my haircut, there's no haircut to see," and I guess they catch on, and I just tell them I can't take my hat off 'cause I'm a cancer patient, and when I tell certain people that, they get nice all of the sudden. They start talking to me in a different way. First they talk to you in a nagging way, then they start talking all nice, like they feel sorry for me or something. I don't go for that though.

———————————

When I came back into school I didn't have any hair and I just told them it was from the treatment that my hair fell out. Because most of them know that because an aunt has cancer, or someone else. It's a very big thing but I liked not having any hair. Actually, it looks better. I had really stiff hair and everything. It's hard to control. It's a lot easier this way. When I had hair I'd be afraid to change it because what would happen if it looked bad. I figure, now I don't have it, and when it grows back, I figure I'll just let it grow in the way I want it to. Just on the top and shave off the sides of it, and just push it back. Sometimes I miss it just 'cause thinking what I could do with it.

You never concede that it's going to happen to you until it starts happening. You always think that you're going to be the person who doesn't lose their hair, 'cause it hasn't happened. And you don't even know whether that's good or bad. You know, if it's supposed to and it doesn't, great, you still have your hair, but is there something wrong with the treatment or what? Fear starts popping up.

Anyway, what happened with me was that as soon as, I don't know how long it was, probably two weeks, I finally woke up with a couple hairs on my pillow, just a couple. And at that time I pretty much knew that it was going to start to fall out. And sure enough, I didn't do anything to my hair then, but it started to come out a little bit at a time. My hair started coming out more and more on my pillow and finally I started actually pulling it out just to speed it up. And when I did that in front of my mother she would really freak out, 'cause you could really take out a huge chunk at a time. She was really frightened by me pulling out my hair that way. I guess it was another sign that I was going through this thing. Everyone would look at me as being sick, as though my hair loss—my mom was probably doing the same thing. She knew it the whole time anyway, she thought it was really, you know, it's really a fact now. I didn't really mind doing that. I knew, I guess I knew that it was supposed to happen, I was kind of happy it was happening because it was supposed to. And it didn't really bother me.

At first my hair didn't change that much, it changed gradually, 'cause this thing didn't happen over a day. It happened over about two weeks. I would look a little bit different. The way I looked would be a little bit different, until finally it got to the point where it was very thin all over, and there were even some parts that were basically bare. And it just went on and on. And I never took a shower above my neck when my hair was coming out. I didn't want to see it all in the drain and all that disgusting stuff. I'd much rather just pull it out, put it in the garbage can, but I saved a little bit, a little tuft.

I wear a cap when I go around to different parts of the hospital because it takes away a lot of the stress. When they see a young person walking or being wheeled around in a wheelchair and you're bald, they immediately associate that with being totally sick. And I really find that unpleasant to be looked at as if I'm totally sick. People stare, normal, everyday people walking down the hall, even sometimes, once in a great while a nurse, but usually it's just people walking by. So I wear a cap and reduce the number of stares I get.

I'm not used to that 'cause all my life I had thick, beautiful hair. Since I was born, I'd say. It used to be real long. And I guess, you know, it was something I got used to, attached to. I knew it was gonna happen, but sometimes I just tried to prevent it, and I'd say, "Oh, it's not going to happen to me." But it did and I just had to get used to it 'cause there was nothing I could do to stop it.

They say that my hair is gonna fall off, but I have confidence my hair is not gonna fall off. I'm gonna come out good. And I guess the doctors don't know about the chemotherapy because you're supposed to stay in the hospital a month and a half, and I'm gonna stay for sixteen days.

*A*dvice for others who have cancer

A child who has cancer enters a special environment that has its own rules of conduct, procedures, and social affiliations. There is an initiation process by which newly diagnosed children come to adapt to this climate. During this period, the advice of other children with cancer is very helpful and often necessary. Those who already are initiated recognize this and willingly offer advice to the novice.

Of all the different kinds of help that other patients can offer, advice regarding how to cope with having cancer and how to adjust to the continuing uncertainties associated with treatment is the most significant. All children who have cancer have their own opinions about the best ways of coping, and sooner or later they all recognize that only another child who has gone through the cancer experience can truly understand what it is like, and therefore such a person assumes the special role of mentor. The advice that these children have for others who have cancer applies not only to other children but to anyone with cancer.

The first thing I think when you get the disease, you have to learn to accept it, because if you don't accept it, then there's like something inside of you fighting for the rest of you 'til it's all over. There's no peace like that. The biggest thing is to learn to accept. If you don't, then you blame other people, you might not treat other people right.

There are certain things you will want to know, but you won't find out unless you ask because people care for one another, that's true, but if you don't show concern for yourself, then there's a lack of care from someone else towards you. This is how I see it. Treating cancer is like a routine to some people, and only some people that try to understand it, try to realize what another person is going through, then can that person relate with the person that has cancer.

Learn how to care for yourself, learn how to be concerned for yourself. It's not that people are not concerned, some people really want to talk, but if you learn how to care for yourself and accept it, then it could really take you through it. But my biggest advice is learn to think about God. I can say that was my consolation when people weren't around, that I had somebody to talk to and not talking to myself because there is a God. It also gives you that peace. With me, I really have to talk with somebody to make them realize where I come from, and what I was mostly glad about was that I knew God before this thing happened to me. A lot of people don't think about Him until something happens to them, that's when you know Him, and that's not bad, but then I would say learn how to pray because people can't always be there for you.

———————

Forget about it, don't have the leukemia inside your head, don't fear death 'cause everybody dies, don't even think about it. When the doctors tell you your leukemia is forty percent curable, don't think about that forty percent, don't think of yourself as a statistic, you're a human being, so don't think about the statistics, don't read the books, don't get scared when the books say you might die, you just go about living your normal life, whatever happens, happens, and when you do get out of the hospital, try to do better things, try to help more than you used to because you're sick and you don't know when your time comes.

Maybe at first, I didn't really have it in my mind like that. Sometimes I would think, "Am I gonna die? What about these blood transfusions with AIDS?" Then you try to tell yourself to forget about all that, because if you start thinking about all of that, it's just gonna make it worse. Maybe it's because they fear death so much, maybe before they were sick they think they were never gonna die, they probably thought they were gonna live until they were ninety, and when they get leukemia they start thinking about death all of the time, I don't think that's gonna help you at all.

For as long as you have cancer, it's gonna be very hard, but there's a light at the end of the tunnel, and you gonna see it, and you gonna be alright and you gonna be cured at the end. But 'til then it's gonna be very hard, you need all the friends and support and family. Don't shy away from what help you can get. Don't try to be macho and don't take help. If you need help getting out of bed, get help, don't try to do it yourself if you can't. Take all the help you can get.

It's gonna be hard as long as you have it. In a way painful because of the chemotherapy, because usually you get sick from it, but everyone reacts differently, so that's one thing. You could have complications from it, and that's hard, and the hospital stays could be long, and they're not very fun, and it's just both hard and annoying. You feel like you can't lead your normal life for a while, you have to put it on hold. Just remember that it's not the end of the world, and keep your hopes up because that's half the battle, you win by thinking that you're gonna win. You gotta think that you're gonna win, then you do win.

Your attitude has to always be up, and you never give up no matter how down you are. You never give up, because if you're so far down and you give up, you're gonna die. But if you keep fighting, you can stay down there until it's over, and then when it's over, go up again. Just saying that, "I have cancer, I'm going to die," there's no reason. The guy that's ready to live is much more happier because he's thinking ahead, he's thinking of what's to come, he's thinking about what's going to happen in the future, he's just thinking of happy things. The other guy just doesn't, he expects to die.

I mean, I always think there's a chance that I'm gonna die. You know, so if everything that they do to me fails, and they say there isn't much hope or whatever, you know, I can sort of face it because I realize that's one of the possibilities, a slim possibility, but it is. But I'm mostly concentrating on that I'm going to fight and live.

You have to try to prepare for like, when you get close to a friend in the hospital and then one day when you come to the hospital, you're told he's not around, 'cause not everybody makes it. You try to prepare just saying that your friend wouldn't want you to give up. Even though he died, he wouldn't like you to give up.

Well, one important thing I think that's real important is that you should never feel ashamed. 'Cause if you feel ashamed then your self-esteem goes down, and you don't have much confidence in the future, you're very pessimistic. You don't think good of yourself and it's no good. I mean, you should not let it come over you like that.

———————

[On telling a new boy friend that you have cancer] Just wait 'til he's able to open up to you. You can tell him what you have, how it happened, you can tell him the whole story then. And just don't be afraid to leave anything out, 'cause I'm sure if he's able to confide in you, you have an understanding between each other. And you can work out arrangements and days you're not feeling well, I'm sure he'll understand and not bother you. 'Cause there were days when I wasn't feeling well and I was like, I don't feel like seeing you today. I would go on these mood swings and it's like, look, I'll get over it but just stay away from me for a couple of days. I'm sure in every relationship there's time, you have to give time for yourself. So I'm sure the girl has to realize that they just can't be together all the time. Give time to yourself and you both can think, you know, what's the next step in your relationship. It's comforting to let everything out.

———————

Don't worry, 'cause there's a lot of doctors that could help you. Let your family support you, and all that. Don't take it that hard 'cause the doctors will take good care of you. Think about good thoughts, don't think about it all the time. Play around, you know, don't think it a lot 'cause then if you think it a lot, it stays in your mind. But if you don't think about it, you think good thoughts, then you'll have a good time.

———————

Have lots of friends to cheer you up. Sometimes a friend cheers me up to play with him, and it really makes me happy but not sad.

Don't try fighting it 'cause it's always going to be there with you. It's always going to be there. Don't like say, "No, no, no," when they come to give you needles and medicine 'cause I tried that and it just doesn't really work. They're gonna still be there, they're not gonna say, "Fine, we're not gonna give it to you," and walk out of the room.

Hold your head up high and just don't let—like, as you go through the treatments, don't let your mind go away to, well, what if I die, and stuff like that. Just think positive 'cause that's the best way to go. And just, as you're going through it, just, um, don't worry about how your friends are gonna react 'cause it may be for some people, your true friends will come out. The ones who will stick by you, the ones who are really your friends will stick by you. And just think to yourself, "I'm gonna go through this as strong as I possibly can."

One of the things I've been learning that's really very important, more and more now, is that you have to remember that it's your life, and people can be very pushy, and you just have to make sure that you're making the decisions in the end. The advice of all the doctors is very good, but you have to decide what you want to do yourself. I was talking to a couple guys who had cancer before, um, and it was interesting to talk to them, because they're cured now. And one of them had it about ten years ago before they had chemotherapy or radiation. And he was told by several doctors that they'd just have to amputate his arm, there was no choice, there was a whole panel of doctors, I don't know if it was at this hospital or another one, but they all told him there's no other choice. And eventually he found my doctor who was just starting, I guess, to do this limb-sparing, which is the kind of operation I'm gonna have. And that's what they ended up doing, and, surprisingly, he's pulled through, he's fine now. But the important thing that he had to say, or the important thing that I got out of what he had to say, was that he made the decision in the end, and everybody tells you this is what we're gonna do, but before you decide anything, you have to make sure that that's what you think is best.

You have to be strong about it. It's not going to be easy, it's gonna be a lot of hard work, and sometimes it's gonna look like everything is going the opposite way from good, going bad, but it will turn out to be good in the end, you just have to be strong. Like when the doctor says do this, you can't say, "No, I'm not gonna take my pills tonight, I'm not gonna do this." You have to do it all the time. You can't say, "I'm not gonna take chemotherapy." You have to do it because it's a life-and-death situation, that's the strong part. It's good to talk about it, not to hide it inside. You can talk to anybody, your parents, family, doctors, social workers, there's also other people you might meet who have the same illness, and you can talk to them too.

I'd tell him how it's really gonna happen. I'd tell him he's got a 50–50 chance to get rid of the cancer or he might have cancer and pass away or something. I'd tell him how it is. I ain't just gonna beat around the bush like the nurse will. The nurse be like, "You're gonna get your chemotherapy, you're gonna get over it, probably in a year's time you'll be out on the street like nothing ever happened." But it's not true, some people get over it and some people don't. Some people can handle the medicine and some people can't, I'm not gonna lie, "You could die from it, anybody could." That's how it is. Don't have nobody to talk to. You always have a friend in the hospital to go talk to, somebody's always going to be around for you here. Stay happy, don't be sad, keep a strong feeling in your heart that your going to get over this. Whatever happens to you, make sure that you know that the doctors are going to try to do the best they can for you. Never underestimate nobody 'cause your going to need somebody there for you.

If you're just another kid who got problems, you'll feel alone 'cause your friends ain't gonna be around with you in the hospital. So make a lot of friends in the hospital. Talk to people who have the same situation. Try not to make yourself like an outcast. And just because you might have a piece of your body taken away from you doesn't mean that, like, you cannot associate with other people, or do things with other people. There's a lot of people that are scared and everything and they think, "Oh, this won't work." But like, keep a good mind functioning, like, always look ahead. 'Cause a lot of kids like me get cured, you know. So it's like, always think positive 'cause there is positive.

I had a friend, and she had passed away from cancer. And like if, if that ever happens to someone, they should just take it well, you know. Like if someone passed away, you know, with like cancer, just take it well. It's not to like, don't get too into it. I'm saying it's OK if you cry, except like don't take it too personally.

Friends and family relations

Cancer poses a variety of stresses on families as well as close friends. The siblings and parents of children who have cancer have special needs, and the children have a special role to play in responding to these needs. In some cases, these stresses disrupt relationships and distance the child with cancer from their family and friends. In most cases, however, relationships are strengthened, and friends and family are brought closer together. Either way, having cancer is a test of these relationships.

My friends help me out a lot, they say "Don't do this, don't do that." Like say you want to go out to a disco, they say you shouldn't go out there because there's a lot of people and with leukemia my defense level is low, so they say that they rather stay home with me. Or like going to the movies, they tell me they'll go with me in the daytime 'cause in the nighttime it's usually packed and it's a closed area. They do a lot of things they wouldn't do if I wasn't sick. They help me out a lot, like sometimes they hang around at my house on Friday nights, and I know they'd rather be doing something else, and one friend will say let's leave, and the rest of them will say, "No, we want to stay with him." They stay in the house watching basketball games, and they won't leave. Sometimes, they won't leave until one in the morning.

One person who I thought wasn't a real good friend 'cause we used to argue a lot was here every day almost. He comes over, calls my house every day. I thought he was my friend, but not as close. He takes me out, drives me around, and he's like a wild guy, but every time he's with me he calms down, and when he takes me out he always asks me if I'm getting sick, how I'm feeling. So you found out who really cares for you and who don't and I feel happy about that.

I see some kids in the hospital, they don't get as much attention, their mothers hardly visit, and when I ordered food out, I used to tell my mother, "Give him some of my allowance money and buy some food for him also 'cause they never bring him food. They don't like the hospital food either, so give him some of that, things he regularly eats." So I help others out too because I see some parents, I never see them here with their kids.

———————————

Everyone's your friend when you're always around, but when you're not around, people that really miss you, always talk to you and are glad to talk to you, and when they see you and stuff are glad to see you and stuff, but the people that say they're your friends and stuff and that don't really keep in contact with you, you can really know that they're not, um, real friends, they don't really care, I guess.

But my best friend, I mean, you'd love him because I can tell that in all that he's done for me that a normal person just wouldn't do out of the ordinary. He's donated blood platelets, anything that I need. He takes off from work which is, you know, money that he'd earn to come and see me. In the hospital, when I'm feeling bad, he takes off and does it. And that's, you know, that's really a friendship, that's it, you know.

———————————

When I went back to school, my friend Roger, he was like talking to me about it, he kept asking me questions. Like we were playing, we were playing tag, and he like lifted up his shirt 'cause he was hot, and I was about to and then I remembered I had a broviac and that I couldn't 'cause then everybody would see, and he said, "Don't lift your shirt up, because then everybody's going to be asking you what's that, what's that." When I had my cancer there were a whole bunch of things I wish I could have done, like lifting up my shirt and like not having anybody asking me and my friend Roger, like he knew what that was like.

Well, I remember one operation after having my second, yeah, I think my second broviac because the first one had gotten infected. No wait, the first one started coming out, so I had to get a new one. And the second one got infected. Well, my father, he just started breaking down and crying. He never really liked the thought of me getting stuff, you know, with the needle or something. I didn't like my father crying and I'll never forget it. Well, I didn't like seeing him crying. I don't have anything against like letting it out. I think that's good, but I just didn't really like to see him crying. 'Cause, it makes me sad that he loves me so much and he can't do anything.

At first I think it was harder on my parents than it was on me, on my father mostly because he is used to seeing me healthy, seeing me exercising, playing baseball, and he found out, I remember the doctors telling him, I heard him when the doctors told him that I had leukemia. He like fell apart and started crying, something I'd never seen because he'd never seen me sick, so it was hard on him. He didn't work for two weeks, he came to my room and sat down and put his head down it was so hard on him. I tried to help, I'd tell him, "Don't worry, I'll be alright." It was really hard on him and my little brother, too.

My little brother, he didn't see me home for three weeks, he come to the hospital and see me sick, and he'd never seen me sick before. He's seen me doing push-ups, having fun on the street playing football. He'd never seen me sick, so I think it was hard on him too. He gained a lot of weight, they thought he was nervous, he started eating a lot at my aunt's house. I don't think he liked asking me questions, he didn't want to like upset me but he asked my aunt questions. Sometimes when I react to the medicine he gets scared, when I start shaking, he gets scared, but after a while when he sees me right again he gets happy.

My father is really the one who took it hardest, my father and my aunt. My aunt, she's dressing in beige, a promise or something like that for God, they have to do something for a year, she's dressing in beige everyday now, and she's always bringing me food and recipes, saying, "This will help out your blood." She's got two kids and a husband she's got to take care of, but she comes to the hospital every day to see me. My mother, she's strong. She comes in with me every time I have a bone marrow test and a spinal tap, she holds my hand, she takes it strong. Some mothers don't like to go in with their kids for the spinal tap because they think it hurts so much they don't like seeing it, but she goes in every time and she takes it.

It brought my whole family closer, like my cousins and my aunts and my uncles, I think they've gotten closer themselves because of my sickness. My aunt and my mother, they seem to get even more along now, always helping each other out, always together. The family on a whole got together closer, not just my parents, the whole family.

My brother talks to me about certain things, but I think he's also pretty optimistic, I don't think he really accepts or thinks about the possibility of my not making it through, he didn't seem to but all the times he talked to me, he would say things he never said before like, "Bobby, I really love you," and stuff like that. Things we always felt but never said. Same thing, I never said to my parents, "I really love you," and it wasn't that I really don't feel it, and now when they've been so supportive and done so many things for me, I feel guilty asking them to do things that I really need them to do sometimes, or if the doctor says I have to eat a lot, and its midnight and I'm hungry, two or three years ago they would have said, "Go to sleep, you'll eat breakfast in the morning," but now they'll get me something. I feel so guilty, even though it's something that really should be done, and so they'll come up before I go to sleep, and I'll say, "Dad, I love you," and these are things I've never said before, and I don't think I would have said it had it not been for something that really made me see it like this.

Well, my best friend, he was like, he get real mad, he starts hitting things. I said, "You gotta calm down, you know." He like took it worse than I did. He punches walls and stuff, he's real angry, slapping books down, stuff like that. But you calm him down and stuff. Then we just, you know, get back in our old routine, we hang out, you know, the way we used to do, that's it. I didn't have to change anything, you know, just do what I do.

I have a boyfriend I've been going out with for a year, and I thought it was important for him to know when we first started going out that I had cancer. I wear a brace on my leg, because they took out a bone and a nerve and I thought that he should know about it so I told him. But it wasn't easy. 'Cause you don't know how to tell it, you know. 'Cause he's never had cancer, you just don't say that. I was scared because I didn't know how he would react, naturally. And I just sat him down and I told him, "There's things that you don't know about me," and I told him that I had cancer, and I'm in remission now, and so far everything's fine, and yes I wear a brace on my leg, and I'll probably have to wear it forever. But I'm normal, you know, I'm not, it's not contagious, you're not going to get anything. It's not something you can get from being with me, and I don't have it any more. We went on for hours and he asked about a hundred questions, "How did it feel, where did it come from, what kind of treatments did you go through, um, could it come back, what happens if it comes back?" And he accepted it.

———

I've been with a best friend for like five years. Over the winter, we wasn't together because I guess we just wasn't getting along, and then he heard about it, but I don't know who by. Now he comes to see me every day. I stopped hanging out with him and I found another friend. But I guess he likes me a lot, and I like him a lot, but we have our differences. You can't push five years of best friends away for just that, so he was kind of upset when he found out but I like him now like a brother. I'm not gonna just throw my friend away and I guess he'll take me back.

*H*ow *cancer has changed me*

Any child who has cancer is changed in a profound way by the experience. These changes are the result of having to confront issues that most children do not deal with until they are well into adulthood. They concern the meaning of life—what it is all about. Questioning of this kind often leads to greater sensitivity for the emotional needs of others. In this respect, cancer can be a very ennobling experience for children. To paraphrase Hemingway, they come out of it stronger in the broken places. One child described his experience of having cancer in this way: "All great men have their setbacks, but overcoming them shows one's greatness."

I feel like it was a test to show me what I was, to show me where I was at, to show me just how strong I was and how much I knew. It teaches you not to judge, not to go upon what somebody else says, but to watch and to realize what life is all about, that not everybody cares for you, but learning to accept it. I learned that everyone is not concerned about you, although there are some people that will show care, but it made me realize that everyone won't love me, and so it makes you a stronger person because you have to learn how to be independent. Like my mother wasn't there all of the time, so I would learn how to do things for myself.

It also teaches you how to accept and not judge people a lot because you went through it, because you're the person sitting down and you have access to a whole bunch of emotions, and you see how people treat one another, and it teaches you how to accept things. You learn how to give people the right attention and treat them right, and then still realize that they wouldn't always treat you that way. It teaches you a whole lot of things. It's almost like something that prepares you for the world, after this is done, then it's like stepping out of a course almost, and then going out and learning how to treat people. It's like they took a little bit of everything in the world and put it in the hospital, so when I get out of this, then I know how to accept people, how to understand them.

I see this as something small, my coming in here, 'cause I've seen things that other people have gone through. I think going through this you might have a lot of self-pity, and you would wonder, but you never really realize how good you have it until you see someone else suffer. Like one day I was in the activity room, and this patient couldn't really do anything for himself, the nurse always had to come, and it made me realize that you can't complain, it's hard, but you have to accept what you go through. When it first happened I really was pretty strong about it, but then when everything was you, everything seems to revolve around you, it makes you feel good about yourself, but sure, people help you but they can't always be there for you, they have to do things, that's when you're by yourself, then there's a feeling of being alone, and then you really see how strong you are, and it's like you just see yourself in this situation and nobody else. There's a lot of wondering to it, no accusing, but you wonder.

It's made me more mature. It's made me think more about how, how precious life is, really. You know, people don't know, you know, when they say, "God I wish I were dead," and stuff like that, they don't know how alive you are until you're on the edge of death. Because I've been there, and you know, I've said that, you know, when I was well, "God, I wish I were dead," or something, and then when I'm at the edge, you think that you said that, but you're fighting so hard that you don't want to give up.

It's made me kind of grant the little things that I have. Like, when I had surgery to my mouth, I couldn't sneeze, I couldn't cough, I couldn't do any of those little things that people don't think are really, you know, you think sneezing is no big deal but it makes you take those little things for life.

I feel I've matured a lot, because of this. Medical terms that you learn, I've picked them up, and I'm able to explain it in an adult manner. And people are like, what are you talking about? And then I have to get in to details and tell them, well, this attacks this, and this is why I got this, and it all happened because of this, and when I'm able to explain it you know, like an adult would, I feel, wow, I feel grown-up. And it's a good feeling.

It made me a person, you know, made me the kind of person that was able to realize their feelings. Some people can go on, you know, years and years in their lives and not know how they feel or how to express their feelings. And I'm able to do that now. Because it brought out a lot of emotions in me, all at once, like fear, anger, depression, and mostly a lot more negative than positive. And I didn't know what to do, and little by little I had to separate those emotions and find out, you know, what was triggering it. And I found out that it was, you know, the cancer, and if it triggers all these emotions at once then I have to find a way to cope with them.

I know how to just deal with them. I don't take out my emotions on anybody, 'cause I feel it's very unfair. I feel that a person that takes out their emotions on people is very selfish. They only think about their own feelings. But I was able to, you know, recognize these feelings and control them, not let them get out of hand and find a way to defeat them.

———

Well, I've been worrying about lots of things. Like this new thing called AIDS. I'm saying, it's going around, people are getting it, it's not like no one's gotten it. It's just like everything's falling apart. Like the world, it's just like I just see the neighborhood. It's just all the crackheads. Yeah. And the question, also, like about having cancer back again. That sort of worries me too.

———

I think I'm a little more friendlier with people, I don't judge them by their color anymore. I used to do that a little, but it changes everybody I guess in a way.

———

I see the people who are sick, you know, you feel a lot more sympathy for them, you know, than I used to. You know, you feel a lot more, I guess, uh, you think a lot more about doing things. When you're young you used to go out and now you don't, I don't. I know people used to drink and stuff you know, and waste away their lives and stuff. And you say, that's useless, why should you do that, there's no sense to that. I guess you just think about life in a whole different view or something. It's hard to explain. It's like, inside, it's different, you know. It's not like, oh it's just, you know, it's just there, something you gotta work for or something. I guess you can think of it like that, just the way you look at life in general.

There's more that you learn about life when you go through a disease, a scary disease, because it's just, it's a whole new different concept about life. I'm in a hospital and out there is a whole world with a lot of people that's not sick, and when I come into the hospital I come into a new world, with sick people, and I gotta react a different way.

There was a time I had some funny stuff about sick people. But now like when I'm with my friends, and they got something funny to say about somebody sick, or poor, or anything like that, I feel bad, 'cause I'll be like, it's wrong to say that. 'Cause I wouldn't want somebody to do it to me. And I'll be telling them, I'll be explaining to them, that they shouldn't do that, 'cause one day you might get sick, and something happen to you, you might get hit by a car, you might not have no leg or something like that. And then people might be messing with you 'cause you only got one leg, now. And you wouldn't want anybody to do that to you.

So you never know what's going to happen to you. I'll be telling them, you don't know what's going to happen to you, so you just leave people alone, 'cause if people ain't bothering you, why should you bother them? That's why I just like, when I go out on the streets I don't bother nobody like I used to, 'cause I used to be bad, and I just changed to like a different person.

Talking about talking about cancer

The thesis of this book is that children need to be able to talk about their cancer experiences, as a way of helping them adjust to the continuing struggles and uncertainties of having cancer. The children's narratives demonstrate that, given appropriate conditions, most children are remarkably candid in how they express themselves. However, for a variety of reasons that are associated with adults' fears and discomforts about cancer-related issues, most children who have cancer are deprived of these opportunities.

For many children, there is a conspiracy of silence about having cancer.[1] Parents, struggling to cope with their own fears about the uncertainties of their child's cancer and the possibility of losing their child, try to protect him or her by denying the frightening biomedical and emotionally stressful problems associated with cancer. Coming to recognize their parents' fears, denials, and adjustment problems, the children—out of respect, concern, and love for them—come to feel that they have to protect their parents by observing the taboo against confronting their parents with their own fears and uncertainties.

Parents often accept their child's reluctance to talk as evidence that their child is being protected and is not afraid of or worried about having cancer and the uncertainties of surviving. When parents act this way, children are left alone with their concerns and are emotionally alienated from their families. They have no one to turn to but their peers in the hospital who have cancer and with whom they establish incredibly intimate relationships. While such relationships are extraordinarily helpful for children, they are not sufficient, particularly when children learn about the inevitable complications, relapses, and death of some of their peers. While children need the support and comfort of their peers who have cancer, they also need those who are a part of their broader culture.

Everyone—from family to members of the treatment team—participates in a conspiracy of silence about cancer to some extent. To whatever degree such conspiracies establish taboos against talking candidly about the problems associated with having cancer, they will cause children serious emotional problems and will significantly interfere with their long-term capacity to cope with having cancer as well as having survived cancer. How children talk about their cancer experiences is an important prognostic indicator of their psychosocial adjustment. Children who refuse to talk to anyone about it and deny that they are afraid and confused by their illness, or are overly hesitant in admitting it to anyone, are at risk for serious adjustment problems. Some children struggle to deny their fears and uncertainties by pretending that having cancer is "nothing, no big deal." Unless such a pretense is unveiled, it can become emotionally overwhelming. When children do not talk about their fears and uncertainties, it does not mean that they are not afraid and uncertain. Their denial and isolation heightens their fears (including fears of dying) and impairs their adjustment.[2]

Some children are hesitant to talk with their families about their problems because they falsely attribute marital discord among their parents and problems of social deviancy and delinquency among their siblings to their having cancer. These children's perceptions of their families' problems is a projection of their own sense of guilt—a way of blaming themselves for having cancer.

Children need help in understanding that they can be a source of support and adjustment for their families by rejecting any kind of conspiracy of silence. They need help in recognizing and acknowledging the fear and discomfort they perceive when talking about their cancer experiences with those that are close to them, and they need help in finding the courage to confront their families and friends.

Sooner or later all children with cancer discover that being able to talk about it helps them cope. Children expressed the need to talk to their families, to their friends, and to their physicians. Some of them talked about how others reacted to their willingness to talk candidly. Although the children expressed the value of talking to adults and siblings about having cancer, they recognized the special value in talking to other children who have cancer and in helping one another struggle to make sense of and find meaning in their experiences. Also, many children worried about whether they were being told the truth when they talked to their parents and physicians, and some felt that they had to corroborate what they were being told. Many children remarked how, in the beginning, people avoided using the word cancer around them.

In trying to capture the variety of ways in which children talk about their experiences of having cancer and to promote healthier ways of interacting with them, I think it is appropriate to conclude in the children's own voices, talking about talking about having cancer.

———

Some people are afraid of talking to me about cancer. Like I spoke to one in particular and she said that the thought ran through her mind like, "You have cancer, I think if I came, I wouldn't know what I would say to you," and she said, "I was thinking most of the time if I went there, I would probably just sit there and look at you," but she said she didn't want to come and have to just look at me. She wanted to talk, but she said, being that I had cancer, "What would I say? I don't want to say the wrong thing, I don't want to hurt you," so she was frightened in that sense, maybe of hurting my feelings or saying the wrong thing.

I think what runs through their minds is now that the person has cancer, they take you as not being the same person anymore. This shows you just exactly who you are, what you can do, how far you can go, and I went through this because really I didn't want to be on the phone that much. At times I just sat down and thought, and I realized that sometimes, that sometimes, I wanted people to call me, I wanted to talk to somebody, anybody, but then sometimes, I didn't want to talk to people I just wanted to think.

When you talk to the doctors, you have to show concern, you have to show that you care about yourself because I feel they told me what they feel I should know, but not as much as I wanted to know. Like I said, I talk a little more now with people and like they would tell me when my treatments would come and what kind of medications I would get, but the thing I wanted to hear was, "How do you feel I will turn out, how do you think the results would come?" They never want to tell you that.

[About telling children the diagnosis] It depends on the age of the kid, how mature he is. I think they should find out first his attitude, they should talk to him first, see how strong he is. If you think he's strong, that he's gonna handle it, then you should tell him the truth, but if you talk to him and you find out that he's too sensitive, that he'll get scared or frightened, then maybe you should hide it from him. Also on how much support he gets, if he's got a strong family behind him and he's a strong kid, then you should tell him straight out the truth because he might find out anyway, and if he finds out, he might get mad if you were trying to hide it. I think you should tell the kid the truth and have somebody talk to him and tell him, "Don't worry about it, just live your life out."

They don't understand what's happening to them and that makes them afraid of chemotherapy because you get sick from it. They think, "He's hurting me, this is hurting me, they're just making me worse, or they're doing this to me because they want to hurt me." They don't understand, I don't think, so it's harder for them. It's probably hard for a lot of people, even the older kids sometimes. But it's good when they tell you things.

Yeah, that's one of the good things because they tell you what's going on, what they're doing, and not that they shouldn't because it's good that they do, because it's your body that they're gonna mess with and just to know what they're doing is good, and before they do it they tell me. There's some people who don't want to know, and for that reason the nurses and doctors won't tell them. If they say, "I don't want to know," they won't tell them, but it's good if you say, "I want to know," and they'll tell you. I like to know what's going on. The doctors, nurses, orthopedic people, they've all told me everything. When I have questions, I ask them. I'm not afraid to just because they're doctors and they have the answers. And they're not worried doesn't mean I'm not worried and don't have questions. I have questions and want to know.

There was a book and some pamphlets that I read and it made sense, now I know what it's like. I'd read them and then

I'd go to the hospital and ask the doctors, "What is this for?" and they'd say exactly what the pamphlet said so then I'd know that they weren't lying to me.

―――――――

I think kids should know everything they can about their cancer. My mother got a book out and part of it was kids talking about it, but they had already been cured from cancer. I think I would feel better if I heard kids talking about it while they still had it because I have it and they have it, and it just makes you feel better to know that. Like if they have questions that they need to be answered that they don't want to ask the doctor or their mother or something. Like, you know, questions about how your friends act and stuff. When you talk to somebody I think it helps a lot. Yea, and I guess, it's nice to know that I could help some other kid too.

―――――――

When I'm stressed, I feel much better just letting it out and not holding it in. If I was to sit and think about it, and let it all get to me, and then think about everything else, and let everything else get to me, I'd go crazy so I'd just tell somebody everything that was going on in my mind. And then I'd feel much better.

―――――――

It's comforting to let everything out. I'm able to now, you know, and I feel good when I talk about it. And like your book, if it was a present to a child just beginning, they should read it. I'm in it, and I give good advice [laughs].

―――――――

I be thinking that like the doctors they be telling me everything. There's one thing I honestly thinking like, when, um, I
used to think that when they be giving me certain medicines,
like they give me a new medicine. I thought that they was
giving me for something I didn't know, and they wasn't telling me something. So that's why when I'm here, I just ask
them why is they giving me this, why this, and because I ask
them 'cause, as they say, "Feel free to ask." So, I just always
ask them to make sure.

I don't feel that they would hold something behind my back
that I shouldn't know 'cause I think I have a right to know.
Like if something's going wrong, I want to know about it and I
want to know why it's going wrong. And if somebody made a
mistake I want to know who did it and how it was done.

It really helps to talk. I'm not sure exactly. I think just to know
that somebody realizes that those feelings are there and to
know they're going to help you to fight them. Because my
mother reassured me that, that we're not alone. And I think
also just to have said it to somebody. Sometimes, when you're
afraid of something, your mind can really play tricks on you
and you start to believe that it's not really there. And to have
said it to somebody else who you respect makes it become
concrete. And you realize it's not such a silly fear, that it is
something you have to deal with. Yeah, so I've learned it's
better to talk in any situation, not just cancer. I don't think
there's a personal airing that could solve all the problems in
life, but certainly there are some that cancer causes and that
might not develop right away. I have a feeling that down the
road there are going to be things that I didn't expect at all.

Just come out straight with them, when you got something to say to them, just come out straight 'cause that's better than beating around the bush and feeling bad thinking that you're going to say something to them that they don't want to hear. So I just think that you should come straight out with what you have to say to 'em. I tell the doctor, if you're gonna say something to me, just tell me straight. Sometimes they beat around the bush, and sometimes they come straight out with what they have to say to me. They'll say something to back up their words that they have to say. They back it up with easier words, a calmer word than it supposed to be. Like they say, if they're trying to say "You got cancer." Alright I've got cancer, that's what I want to hear, but they be like, "You got this certain thing that you'll get over in so much time." They won't come straight out, they say another word for this type of cancer, but they never said cancer.

I didn't know I had cancer until I asked my mother what it was. She said I got this other disease, but they ain't never said it was cancer. My mother had to tell me it was cancer. That's wrong. That's like lying.

———————————

Talk to others, that's the best thing to do. Yeah, you get to know people. Like this one guy he was in the treatment and we talked 'cause I had gone in before him, right? I told him a lot of things that happened, you know, I told him a lot of things that happened, like, when I was on the treatment, a lot of things. You know, he started listening. He just sat and listened. He's not the type of person that's like, "I don't want to hear this, I don't want to hear this, I don't want to hear that." He just sat and listened to me, you know. And we became friends, you know. We're real close now, we know each other like, I don't know, we know each other like a year now. It's like we knew each other all our life. You know, 'cause I know him real good and now he knows me real good. And he knows what I'm going through, and I know what he's going through.

Some patients they don't want to be bothered 'cause they're scared. They stay in their room, you know, I'm not gonna go in there after you. You know, come out, be a part of the crowd, you know, we'll go in a group. They don't want to go in a group. 'Cause they got cancer, they don't want to be bothered. Come out, be a part of life, you know. You'll probably going to go in there and talk to them and they'll probably listen, but they probably wouldn't really be paying attention to you. You'll probably just be sitting there talking to them with the TV on.

That's like, that's how it is like, you know, I was talking to this guy about, I was telling this guy about my broviac. He didn't want to hear it. He didn't want to hear that. I know he didn't. He was so scared he was going to get a broviac, or anything, he didn't want to hear about it, he didn't want to hear what I had to say then. Like, I don't know, I probably don't know if I would have did the same thing, but you know, I didn't.

———

You gotta be with people. You gotta talk to people, get out your emotions and your frustrations by talking to someone else. If you keep everything inside it's no good. Everything gets worse.

———

Kids, they get courage from each other. It means everything. Like, if another guy got leukemia, he just got it, you go up to him and say, like, "I've been through it, don't worry, you'll be fine," you can tell him. It will be hard at first, but then he'll get better. I'd tell him the truth that it's painful, the spinal tap and bone marrows and all that. You get scared when you see all these needles and stuff, like sometimes they can't find your veins and they just poke you and poke you, and you can't do anything. And it's OK to be afraid and don't hold it in. Tell your doctors, tell them how you feel, tell them that you're afraid. If you hold it in, you'll get depressed thinking about it, all you think about is being afraid. Talk to anybody, your parents, anybody, friends, anybody who'll listen.

Afterword

Working with children
who have cancer

In getting to know the members of pediatric oncology treatment teams, including physicians, nurses, social workers, pediatric psychologists, child-life specialists, and administrative assistants, I came to appreciate the uncommon kinds of stresses, frustrations, disappointments, and rewards that come with this kind of professional service. I also learned to appreciate their need to be able to separate themselves from their work when they are not on service as much as their need to share with their colleagues, while on service, the anguish and fallibility that they often feel in the presence of children's suffering.

Hospitals provide many different kinds of institutional props and defense mechanisms, including medical jargon and grim humor, to help their staff cope with—and often at times to deny—their feelings about their patients so as to focus on the strictly medical aspects of illness.[1] However, in the world of pediatric oncology, one is struck by how much these institutional props are dismissed. More than specialists in any other branch of medicine, pediatric oncologists stay in touch with their feelings for their patients and share them with their colleagues. In this way, they are better able to respond to the emotional needs of their patients when considering treatment decisions.

This was readily apparent during the pediatric oncology staff conferences I attended. Often there was as much commentary about the emotional state of patients as there was about their medical condition. During a typical case conference in which the status of each patient is reviewed and treatment decisions are made, I noted the following comments about the patient's (and sometimes their parents' and the staff's) psychological reactions and emotional needs:

He's not even depressed because of the cancer, he's depressed because he can't walk without a cane and a walker. *Physician*

I can't tell if he wants to tune me out or he's so drugged that . . . *Nurse*

He cried with me a lot. How scared he was, he never thought about dying, he really felt helpless. *Nurse*

She was frightened to death at being in the recovery room. *Nurse*

He has a low anxiety threshold. *Physician*

Without his family this kid would collapse. *Chief of service*

Basically, what she was telling us is that, "I don't want to know." *Chief of service*

She's had a personality transformation. *Chief of service*

She's really missing her mom and she's really verbal about it. *Nurse*

She's another mother who lets her own kid go through this whole procedure alone. *Chief of service*

He likes being accepted by the other kids. *Social worker*

He gives strength to everybody he talks to. *Nurse*

He said he wasn't scared when he had the relapse but now he's very, very scared. *Nurse*

I'm frightened to send him home. *Chief of service*

I hope it's just denial and not . . . *Chief of service*

I spoke to both of them and scared the hell out of them [in response to the parents not showing up for appointments with the staff and leaving their child alone in the hospital]. *Chief of service*

I think we need to spend more time with the family. *Physician*

He's a tough-as-nails kid but he was so frightened. It's nice to see him frightened because he's just a nine-year-old kid and doesn't need to be so worldly wise. *Chief of service*

She has a pathological fear of blood drawing. *Chief of service*

She's such a brave girl, she hardly complains at all. The mother's just having a hard time. She doesn't talk to anyone. *Nurse*

A lot of the barriers are down [referring to a father finally feeling comfortable enough to be able to play with his son again]. *Physician*

I think the danger in her case is psychological [referring to a patient's reaction to a delay in her treatment]. *Physician*

I think we have to listen to how the family feels about this. *Physician*

Many other issues regarding the emotional status of patients were discussed during this particular case conference. For example, the question was raised whether the hospital could assume the costs for overseas long-distance phone calls so that a patient could talk to her mother once a week. There was concern about a Black teenager's reaction to the regrowth of his hair, which was coming in "straight." In another case a nurse volunteered on her own time to take a mother to get her nails done as a way of boosting the mother's sagging morale now that her son had entered intensive care. The staff discussed what to do about a mother who needed to be in a drug treatment program and who was not bringing her young child to the hospital when appropriate. They also discussed hospital translators, who were editing and distorting their speech to non-English-speaking parents and patients, including avoiding words like "death" and "dying." A medical resident was criticized for asking a six-year-old patient if she wanted medication to relieve her pain instead of making that judgment for the child, and questions were asked about why another young child was left alone in a surgery recovery room. The staff discussed how to set limits for a father who was physically abusing his son and how to explain to a sexually active adolescent the danger of her becoming pregnant while on chemotherapy. The decision was made to release special funds to buy some new clothes for an impoverished patient who was beginning to lose his hair, so that he might feel better about himself. These kinds of concerns transcended the strictly medical condition of patients, but they were routinely discussed during case conferences and were recognized simply as an essential component of competent medical practice in pediatric oncology.

How do they cope?

When I described to people outside the pediatric oncology profession the kind of book I was preparing, they often asked me what the people are like who choose to work with children who have cancer, why they choose to do it, and how they cope. I do not think that there is any one kind of special or exemplary person that chooses to enter this kind of work. It certainly is not a spiritual calling, and it does not necessarily reflect an uncommon type of character or disposition. Each person has his or her own reasons for wanting to work with children who have cancer.

People who work with these children assume special roles in their patient's lives and value their patient's gratitude. They share hope and reassurance with their patients, without minimizing the limitations of medicine. They learn how to relate to the normal developmental needs, frustrations, and achievements of these children. The experienced ones have learned how to abstain from taking their practice home with them so that the everyday concerns of their friends and families do not appear trivial compared with the problems their patients confront.

When I first began meeting with children who had cancer, it was always on a Thursday. I thought that I was handling my emotions fairly well until I began to realize that friends or family would always find excuses to avoid being with me on Thursday evenings. When I recognized this pattern and asked some of them about it, even those who had not been aware of how I was spending those particular days told me that I appeared different to them on Thursday evenings. I was more impatient, edgy, and irritable, often intolerant of others, and more prone than usual to be provoked.

I then realized that it was important to get help in dealing with this behavior, so I began meeting with one of my former therapy supervisors. During our meetings I began to discern how much I was identifying with these children who had cancer and how much I was experiencing and acting out in an empathic, yet inappropriate, way their anger, frustration, and need to assign blame. I had to work through these reactions emotionally in therapy supervision; simply being intellectually aware of their source and the symptomatic processes that led to their expression was not adequate.

Whenever I tell this story to members of pediatric oncology treatment teams, they tell me very similar stories of their own. These conversations have lead me to appreciate that people who work with children who have cancer need to seek help in dealing with these very personal kinds of stress. The help can come either individually or in a group as part of in-service training programs. Getting some kind of therapeutic help is particularly important for those of us who have not had cancer ourselves because we are more prone to overidentify with these children and to unwittingly want to assume their burdens for them.

In the same way that all children who have cancer at some time pose the question "Why me?" we inevitably ask "Why them?" and "Why this particular child?" In our culture, adults feel compelled to protect and honor the future of children. This attitude is reflected in the popular idiom that any kid in America can grow up to be President; it is tormenting for us to recognize the more likely scenario, which is that any kid in America can die of cancer. Because the "Why me?" and "Why him or her?" kinds of questions have no answers, we must come to terms with the feelings that generate them, or else we will endlessly search for answers everywhere, and our feelings, so displaced, will spill out on everyone.

The emotional reactions of those who work with children who have cancer are similar in some ways to the reactions of parents and siblings of a child who has cancer. However, for the family, these emotions are constrained to a single child, and they are relatively time-limited. The child in time will either recover or die from his or her illness. If the child recovers, family members will feel relief and will have opportunities to see their son or daughter or sibling resume the normal tasks of growing up (although the experience of having had cancer will never be fully resolved for the child or the family). If the child dies, there will be intense mourning for the loss. In either case these natural processes usually allow family members to release and resolve the anger and frustration that come from identification with their child or their brother or sister.

There is no natural process of release and resolution for members of pediatric oncology teams. Unless their anger, frustration, and uncertainty are therapeutically resolved, these emotions will be renewed and fortified with each new patient. The successful resolution is not to become immune to these emotions, to deny them, nor to displace them, but to acknowledge them and their source so that they can be shared within the context of medical practice. Those who fail to do so either become so emotionally overwhelmed by their work that they burn out and prematurely leave their practice, or they become so dispassionate and implacable that their practice is severely impaired.

Notes

Preface

The "number-crunching" study referred to is D. Bearison and C. Pacifici, "Children's event knowledge of cancer," *Journal of Applied Developmental Psychology* 10 (1989): 469–486.

Introduction

1. In 1961, 90 percent of American physicians responded in a survey that they preferred not telling cancer patients their diagnoses. In 1977, 97 percent indicated a preference for telling cancer patients their diagnoses; see D. H. Novack, R. Plumer, R. L. Smith, H. Ochitill, G. Morrow, and J. M. Bennett, "Changes in physicians' attitudes toward telling the cancer patient," *Journal of the American Medical Association* 241 (1979): 897–900. Although oncologists in Africa, France, Hungary, Italy, Japan, Portugal, and Spain indicated that less than 40 percent of their colleagues would use the word cancer with their patients, 90 percent of them reported an increasing trend in their respective countries toward more open disclosure of cancer diagnoses, and most felt that revealing a diagnosis of cancer to patients would have a positive effect in terms of their coping, compliance, and tolerance of treatment; see J. Holland, N. Geary, A. Marchini, and S. Tross, "An international survey of physician attitudes and practice in regard to revealing the diagnosis of cancer," *Cancer Investigation* 5 (1987): 151–154.
2. C. Binger, A. Albin, R. Feuerstein, J. Kushner, S. Zoger, and C. Mikelsen, "Childhood leukemia: emotional impact on patient

and family," *New England Journal of Medicine* 280 (1969): 414–418. D. Adams, *Childhood Malignancy: The Psychosocial Care of the Child and His Family* (Springfield, MA: Charles C. Thomas, 1979). G. Koocher and J. E.O'Malley, *The Damocles Syndrome: Psychological Consequences of Surviving Childhood Cancer* (New York: McGraw-Hill, 1981).

3. J. Katz, *The Silent World of Doctor and Patient* (New York: Free Press, 1984).

4. See, for example, L. LeShan, *You Can Fight for Your Life: Emotional Factors in the Causation of Cancer* (New York: M. Evans & Co., 1977). Studies of this kind describe a general personality type among cancer patients that supposedly precedes their development of cancer. Those with "cancer-prone personalities" are said to have had a childhood marked by chronic feelings of social alienation and depression, and to have suffered from the traumatic loss of meaningful relationships. Despite the often sensationalized accounts in the media about these kinds of findings, there currently is no reliable evidence to support the existence of socioemotional conditions in childhood that would predispose individuals to acquiring cancer. See B. H. Fox, "Premorbid psychological factors as related to cancer incidence," *Journal of Behavioral Medicine* 1 (1978): 45–117. K. Dusynski, J. Shaffer, and C. Thomas, "Neoplasm and traumatic events in childhood: are they related?" *Archives of General Psychiatry* 38 (1981): 327–331.

5. See D. Bearison and C. Pacifici, "Psychological studies of children who have cancer," *Journal of Applied Developmental Psychology* 5 (1984): 263–280, for a comprehensive review of research about the adjustment problems of children who have and who survive cancer.

6. E. H. Waechter, "Children's awareness of fatal illness," *American Journal of Nursing* 71 (1971): 1168–1172. J. J. Spinetta, D. Rigler, and M. Karon, "Anxiety and the dying child," *Pediatrics* 52 (1973): 841–845. L. Zeltzer, J. Kellerman, L. Ellenburg, J. Dash, and D. Rigler, "Psychosocial effects of illness on adolescence. Part II: Impact of illness on crucial issues and coping styles," *Journal of Pediatrics* 97 (1980): 132–138. D. Schuler, A. Polcz, T. Revesz, R. Koos, M. Bakos, and N. Gal, "Psychological late effects of leuke-

mia in children and their prevention," *Medical and Pediatric Oncology* 9 (1981): 191–194.

7. J. J. Spinetta and L. Maloney, "Death anxiety in the outpatient leukemic child," *Pediatrics* 56 (1975): 1034–1037.

8. J. E. O'Malley, G. Koocher, D. Foster, and L. Slavin, "Psychiatric sequelae of surviving childhood cancer," *American Journal of Orthopsychiatry* 49 (1979): 94–96. Koocher and O'Malley, *Damocles Syndrome* (1981). R. K. Mulhern, A. L. Wasserman, A. G. Friedman, and D. Fairclough, "Social competence and behavioral adjustment of children who are long-term survivors of cancer," *Pediatrics* 83 (1989): 18–25.

9. L. Slavin, J. O'Malley, G. Koocher, and D. Foster, "Communication of the cancer diagnosis to pediatric patients: impact on long-term adjustment," *American Journal of Psychiatry* 139 (1982): 179–183.

10. D. Bearison and H. Zimiles, *Thought and Emotion* (Hillsdale, NJ: Erlbaum, 1986). C. Izard, J. Kagan, and R. Zajonc, eds., *Emotion, Cognition and Behavior* (New York: Cambridge University Press, 1984).

11. E. Susman, A. Hollenbeck, E. Nannis, and B. Strope, "A developmental perspective on psychological aspects of childhood cancer," in J. Schulman and M. Kupst, eds., *The Child with Cancer* (Springfield, IL: C. C. Thomas, 1980). J. J. Spinetta and L. J. Spinetta, *Living with Childhood Cancer* (St. Louis: C. V. Mosby, 1981). M. Chesler and O. Barbarin, *Childhood Cancer and the Family: Meeting the Challenge of Stress and Support* (New York: Brunner/Mazel, 1987).

12. Binger et al., "Childhood leukemia" (1969). M. Bluebond-Langner, *The Private Worlds of Dying Children* (Princeton: Princeton University Press, 1978).

13. B. Glaser and A. Strauss, *Awareness of Dying: A Study of Social Interaction* (Chicago: Aldin, 1965). Bluebond-Langner, *Private Worlds* (1978).

14. Katz, *Silent World* (1984).

They only understand what I tell them

1. A broviac is a semipermanent intravenous tube connected to one of the large blood vessels. The other end remains exposed as it

exists the chest wall and is used to withdraw blood and to administer fluids and medication.

Talking about talking about cancer

1. C. Binger, A. Albin, R. Feuerstein, J. Kushner, S. Zoger, and C. Mikelsen, "Childhood leukemia: emotional impact on patient and family," *New England Journal of Medicine* 280 (1969): 414–418. M. Bluebond-Langner, *The Private Worlds of Dying Children* (Princeton: Princeton University Press, 1978).
2. J. Vernick and M. Karon, "Who's afraid of death on a leukemia ward?" *American Journal of Diseases of Children* 109 (1965): 393–397.

Afterword

1. R. Fox, *Experiment Perilous: Physicians and Patients Facing the Unknown* (Glencoe, IL: Free Press, 1959).